Lecture Notes on Psychiatry

By James Willis

Drug Dependence
Faber & Faber 1969

Addicts, Drugs and Alcohol Re-examined
Pitman 1973

Clinical Psychiatry
Blackwell Scientific Publications 1976

Drug Use and Abuse
Faber & Faber 1989

Lecture Notes on Psychiatry

JAMES WILLIS
MB FRCP(Edin.), FRCPsych, DPM
Formerly Head, Division of Psychiatry,
King Faisal Specialist Hospital
and Research Centre,
Riyadh, Saudi Arabia;
Formerly Consultant/Psychiatrist,
Guy's Hospital, London;
King's College Hospital,
London;
and Bexley Hospital,
Kent

J. A. MARKS
MB ChB(Edin.), MRCPsych
Consultant Psychiatrist,
Halton General Hospital,
Runcorn, Cheshire

SEVENTH EDITION

OXFORD

BLACKWELL SCIENTIFIC PUBLICATIONS

LONDON EDINBURGH BOSTON

MELBOURNE PARIS BERLIN VIENNA

© 1964, 1968, 1972, 1974, 1979, 1984,
  1989 by
Blackwell Scientific Publications
Editorial Offices:
Osney Mead, Oxford OX2 0EL
25 John Street, London WC1N 2BL
23 Ainslie Place, Edinburgh EH3 6AJ
3 Cambridge Center, Cambridge,
  Massachusetts 02142, USA
54 University Street, Carlton
  Victoria 3053, Australia

Other Editorial Offices:
Arnette SA
2, rue Casimir-Delavigne
75006 Paris
France

Blackwell Wissenschaft
Meinekestrasse 4
D-1000 Berlin 15
Germany

Blackwell MZV
Feldgasse 13
A-1238 Wien
Austria

First published 1964
Reprinted 1966
Second Edition 1968
Reprinted 1970
Third Edition 1972
Fourth Edition 1974
Reprinted 1976
Fifth Edition 1979
Portuguese Edition 1980
Sixth Edition 1984
Seventh Edition 1989
Reprinted 1991

Set by Times Graphics, Singapore;
printed and bound in Great Britain
by Billings and Sons Ltd, Worcester

DISTRIBUTORS

Marston Book Services Ltd
PO Box 87
Oxford OX2 0DT
(*Orders*: Tel: 0865 791155
        Fax: 0865 791927
        Telex: 837515)

USA
  Mosby-Year Book, Inc.
  11830 Westline Industrial Drive
  St Louis, Missouri 63146
  (*Orders*: Tel: (800) 633-6699)

Canada
  Mosby-Year Book, Inc.
  5240 Finch Avenue East
  Scarborough, Ontario
  (*Orders*: Tel: (416) 298-1588)

Australia
  Blackwell Scientific Publications
  (Australia) Pty Ltd
  54 University Street
  Carlton, Victoria 3053
  (*Orders*: Tel: (03) 347-0300)

British Library
Cataloguing in Publication Data
Willis, James, *1928–*
  Lecture notes on psychiatry — 7th ed.
  1. Man. Mental disorders
  I. Title   II. Marks, J.A.
  616.89

  ISBN 0-632-02452-6

In loving memory of
MURIEL WILLIS
1929–1984
and
ZOË RUTH MARKS
1975–1985

Contents

Preface

To me has fallen the honour of co-authoring and editing the 7th edition of Dr James Willis's *Lecture Notes on Psychiatry*. This has proved the most popular of a popular series and I have therefore kept the style and content of previous editions, merely updating where necessary. Chapter 5 on neuroses and personality disorders has been expanded to provide a conceptual model for what many students (and qualified doctors) find a vague and difficult field. This has its merits and demerits, but at least offers a 'bone' for students to chew over their ideas on how to look at human character. I am especially grateful to Dr Neil Simpson of Manchester Royal Infirmary for Chapter 8, to my colleague, Dr Margaret Bamforth, for Chapter 9, and to Dr James Higgins of the Mersey Regional Forensic Psychiatry Service for advice on Chapter 11. Finally, the inspiration of Dr Willis's previous editions runs throughout the book and he has directly assisted me with advice and criticism, including the contribution of the chapter on eating disorders.

John Marks

An Introduction to Psychiatry

Medical students often say that they find psychiatry interesting but disappointing. Interesting because psychiatry is a clinical subject and all students seem to like this, disappointing because, as they frequently put it, 'it all seems vague and woolly'; also they are put off by the apparent lack of a sound body of psychiatric knowledge and the disagreements about diagnosis and treatment.

This book is not intended as a comprehensive text; the length and omissions should make that clear. It is written to try and answer the sort of questions that students seem to need answering fairly quickly when they start a psychiatric clerkship. They find themselves in difficulties because they have to learn a new language and acquire a new set of concepts of illness if they are to retain any interest in psychiatry at all. Too often they are discouraged from trying and emerge as doctors with blind spots for psychological illness.

The training of medical students remains a subject for discussion, research and revision but as yet it does not adequately prepare the majority of students for much more than a somewhat unwary first encounter with the practice of psychiatry. Students tend to have heard that psychiatry is a discipline 'by schisms rent asunder' and this may make them unnecessarily sceptical, particularly if their half notions are reinforced by the misinformation still so freely available from an intriguing range of sources.

Also there *are* unresolved dilemmas about what things should be taught. Certain medical schools may favour a clinical approach based on traditional diagnosis, treatment and prognosis. Others favour early introduction of the student to psychological principles—showing how human behaviour may be governed by unconscious processes and relating this to interpersonal relationships and *their* consequences in people's life styles and behaviour. Whilst others have suggested that students need to be introduced quite early to the practice of psychotherapy—since this will provide them with a living illustration of human psychopathology. But while these divisions of opinions may exist (since as yet no one has *proved* what the needs of students are), at least we see the beginnings of a medical student training in which the importance is stressed of the patient as an individual and as a social being—not a mere collection of mechanical systems.

Medical student training may be the subject of discussion, research and revision, but the fact is that it does not equip students for the easy assimilation of psychiatric attitudes and ideas.

For a start the student finds it necessary to re-examine his or her own concept of disease. Up to now he or she has had no difficulty in seeing that patients with tumours, fractures, diabetes, etc. are in diseased states. The psychiatric patient, on the other hand, often appears well and disclaims symptoms; no handicap is obvious until it is found that the patient's inner life is dominated by a series of fantastic beliefs which have caused an alteration in life style so that he or she is now in hospital—maybe against his or her will. What can be made of that? Is the patient ill? Are there many patients like that and if so what is wrong with them?

Psychiatry deals with this sort of patient and many others; what they all have in common is disturbances affecting their behaviour, emotions, thinking and perception. Perhaps most important of all is the recognition that 'psychiatric illness' occurs when these disturbances are real changes which persist and exceed commonly accepted limits of normality and are changes about which the patient may complain, be bothered and puzzled about—so that we are justified in regarding them as symptoms. This is the psychiatric frame of reference. We can set it down more formally by saying that we recognize psychiatric illness by examining the patient's

1 behaviour;
2 mood;
3 perception;
4 thought content;
5 intelligence level
6 memory
7 concentration   } cognitive functions;
8 orientation in space and time

and by discerning abnormalities make a clinical diagnosis.

The manifestations of psychiatric disorder can be recognized without great difficulty. The medical student's difficulty in examining psychiatric patients can be traced to:

1 lack of method; and
2 lack of practice.

It is our intention in this work to provide a simple clinical guide to psychiatric language and syndromes.

The student should always remember

1 to listen carefully;
2 to record conscientiously;
3 to avoid interpreting and speculating about what he or she supposes the patient means;
4 to get a history from as many informants as possible; and
5 only to use words that he or she understands.

Classification of mental illness

The ideal classification would be based on aetiology. In psychiatry this is rarely possible except in certain organic disorders (e.g. GPI, delirium tremens), so that classification tends to be descriptive, that is to say based on the dominant observable features of the syndrome (e.g. anxiety, depression). This is unsatisfactory but inevitable at present. The danger of the descriptive method lies in the possibility that the name given to a syndrome may assign to it a separate existence. For example we may talk about schizophrenia without assuming that there is a 'thing' schizophrenia. If the word is allowed to assume a concrete reality this stifles further enquiry.

Classification then may be unsatisfactory but necessary since we have to achieve some sort of order. Many systems are used, some are more satisfactory than others. In this work we will use the following classification: it is clinical, oversimple no doubt, but adequate.

1 Affective disorders:
   depressive states;
   unipolar and bipolar affective disorder.
2 Schizophrenia:
   simple;
   hebephrenic;
   catatonic;
   paranoid.
3 Organic syndromes:
   delirium and subacute delirium;
   dementia.
4 Neuroses:
   anxiety;
   hysteria;
   obsessional disorder;
   hypochondriasis.
5 Personality disorder:
   abnormal personality;
   psychopathy.
6 Mental handicap (mental impairment).

Chapter 1
The History—Some Terms Defined—
The Examination

Introduction

The psychiatric history, like any other, is an attempt to set down an accurate account of an illness. It is taken in the usual way but the technique should be modified to permit the patient to tell his or her story without becoming unnecessarily distressed. Distress and misery are commonplace since the history so often refers to painful topics. The patient should be allowed to start off at any point in the history rather than adhering to a rigid scheme of questioning—there should be time to sort out all the data afterwards.

The first interview

One should attempt to take as full a history as possible on this occasion but it may not be a practical, nor a humane, possibility. This first interview is likely to be an event of great significance for the patient, who may have been dreading it or preparing for it for days and is likely to remember it when it is over. With this in mind, the doctor should do everything possible to make the experience bearable for the patient and resist the temptation to question like a cross-examining attorney.

How to elicit a history

Students often complain that they do not know what questions to ask the patient and are surprised when a more skilled examiner unearths facts they have missed. The answer to this difficulty is relatively simple. A history, after all, is only an edited series of answers to an elaborate and unstructured questionnaire, and with practice the expert learns what questions to ask, and constructs his or her own questionnaire. Listening to others taking a history illustrates this very well—actually this is as good a way of learning to take a history as any, and is not used widely enough.

Symptoms and signs

Modes of presentation and symptomatology are of a different order in psychiatry, though not inevitably so. One patient complains of bodily symptoms, another brings a story of persecution by others, whilst a third complains of altered mood and poor concentration. Many patients have no complaint at all and deny all symptoms, the history being given by relatives, who tell a different story.

The relationship

The relationship between doctor and patient starts as the patient comes through the door. The patient's initial greeting may be friendly, hostile, suspicious or just neutral. Whatever it is, the doctor stands to lose or gain a great deal by his or her

1

own behaviour. There is no substitute for *friendly politeness* and no place for patronizing pseudo-omniscience. Patients should be accepted as they are and not subjected to value judgements. The talkative patient should be permitted to tell his or her story freely at first, and then be guided through areas that the doctor wants to cover so that a comprehensive history can be taken. The reticent patient needs encouragement and although this can be difficult, one must not put words into the patient's mouth.

The place of history taking in diagnosis

There is a fashionable tendency for some psychiatrists to decry diagnosis, to question the 'medical model' of psychiatric illness; and there is good sense in many such criticisms. Just because someone consults a psychiatrist does not automatically confer on that person the status of being ill. This needs to be mentioned, for some psychiatrists talk as if they believed it were the case! Practical psychiatry should remain a clinical subject in which traditional medical training in diagnosis, etc. are of clear usefulness without being overvalued. The clinical approach remains, to date, a humane and pragmatic one. We should recognize too that the clinician always has to be aware of how individual, psychological and social forces may influence the content of an illness but not the form of clinical syndromes—and form is what diagnosis is about. Perhaps we would do well always to remember the large gaps in our knowledge and resist the temptation to conceal them with all-embracing theories which illuminate all and clarify nothing save their continued existence as untested and untestable hypotheses— ugly white elephants which retain our mistakes long after we have forgotten them.

Diagnosis is made by examination of the mental state. The history contributes to our understanding of the mental state—it is a pointer to the diagnosis. History taking takes time. One cannot learn much about a patient in 5 minutes or even 50, for that matter. There is no place in good psychiatry or good medical practice for the 'spot diagnosis'—in psychiatry it generally turns out to be no diagnosis at all. Most diagnostic errors can be traced to poor history taking.

A scheme for history taking

A formal scheme has to be used for writing down the history. This does not mean that one has to take it down in the order that follows.

Complaint

This should consist merely of a short statement of the patient's complaint, or if there is none, a short statement of the reason for his referral for psychiatric opinion.

Family history

In this, one should enumerate the *parents* and *siblings*, noting carefully such details as *ages, employment, illnesses* and *causes of death*. It should also include, where possible, some account of the incidence of any *familial psychiatric illnesses*. Direct questions should always be asked about incidence in the family of epilepsy, delinquency, alcoholism and drug use, and suicide and attempted suicide. The family history too should give some information about the *social status and inter-personal relationships* within the family.

Personal history

This should commence with a note of the date and place of birth. Any information available about the patient's infant development should be recorded with particular reference to *health* during childhood, *neurotic symptoms* and *infant milestones*. *School records* should next be noted down, concentrating not only on facts such as the names of the schools and the leaving age, but attempting if possible to state the individual's attainments at school and to estimate his or her social popularity, etc. *Occupations* should next be considered in chronological order with wages earned and status. These details may throw some light on the person's pre-morbid personality and also on the evolution of the illness since frequently work performance is impaired by psychiatric illness—it may be the presenting complaint, e.g. 'can't seem to cope with my job . . . keep having to change my job . . . can't settle to anything'. It is also useful to make some note of the individual's relationships with employers and colleagues.

Menstrual and psychosexual history

This includes the usual menstrual history with the addition of psychosexual topics such as how the patient acquired sexual information, his or her *varieties* and *frequency* of sexual practice and *fantasy*. The marital history should be noted with details of *engagement, marriage* and *pregnancies* and their outcome. There should always be careful enquiry about psychiatric disturbance during and after pregnancy.

Past illnesses

Recorded chronologically with details of any admissions and treatments received.

Past psychiatric illnesses

Recorded chronologically.

Pre-morbid personality

An attempt should be made to describe as accurately as possible the individual's personality before the illness. This usually causes great difficulty since methods of describing the personality are so imperfect. In practice, the most helpful descriptions of the pre-morbid personality are not those which consist merely of one or two adjectives but rather those which give a portrait of the individual, consisting of a few paragraphs.

Description of present illness

This should be a detailed chronological account of the illness from the onset to the present time. There should always be an accurate description of the order, mode and speed of change in the person's symptomatology.

The psychiatric examination

The examination of the patient does not stop short at the examination of the mental state but includes a general physical examination, and where needed, physical investigation. Many individuals referred to a psychiatrist turn out to have either associated physical disease or else disease causing their altered mental state. Examples of the latter would be such conditions as cerebral tumours, general paresis, disseminated sclerosis and myxoedema. The physical examination, too, has a positive value in the reassurance of a hypochondriacal patient.

Psychiatric language—a few terms defined

Before going any further into details of how we examine and describe the mental state, here is a list of commonly used psychiatric terms.

Anxiety

A feeling of fear or apprehension commonly accompanied by autonomic disturbance. Anxiety may be felt by healthy subjects in the face of stress such as examinations, but is described as morbid anxiety when it pervades the mental life of an individual.

Depression

Pathological mood disturbance resembling sadness or grief. Depression is described as reactive when it can be related to an apparent causal agent and endogenous when it appears out of the blue. The mood change is accompanied by characteristic disturbance of sleep, energy and thinking.

Dementia

Progressive, irreversible intellectual impairment. Dementia is caused by organic brain disease.

Delirium

An organic mental state in which altered consciousness is combined with psychomotor overactivity, hallucinosis and disorientation.

Depersonalization

A subjective feeling of altered reality of the self, e.g. 'I'm not myself any more. I feel as if I were dead; I feel unreal. Different from what I was. If only I could wake up.'

Derealization

A subjective feeling of altered reality of the environment, e.g. 'Everything around me seems strange like in a dream. Things don't look or feel the same.' This is usually associated with depersonalization.

Delusion

A false belief which is inappropriate to an individual's sociocultural background and which is held in the face of logical argument. True delusions commonly have a paranoid colouring (q.v.) and are held with extraordinary conviction. Delusion is thus a primary and fundamental experience in which incorrect judgements are made. The experience of delusion proper precedes its expression in words and hence, when stated, is incomprehensible and beyond argument, e.g. 'I was walking along the street and saw a dog and immediately I knew by the way it stood that I was a special person predestined to save mankind.'

Delusional ideas

Delusional ideas differ from true or primary delusions in that instead of arising out of the blue they occur against a background of disturbed mood and are entirely explicable in that context. Thus the severe delusional ideas of guilt and condemnation and persecution shown by a psychotic depressive are seen to be an outgrowth of the depressive state. In the same way the delusional notions of grandeur and exaltation of the manic spring from his elevated mood—a mood which brings with it breezy overconfidence and insouciance which can easily develop into ideas of omnipotence.

Flight of ideas

Accelerated thinking, characteristically seen in hypomanic and manic illness. The associations between ideas are casual, and are determined by such things as puns and rhymes. However, links are detectable and the flight can be followed.

Hallucinations

A perception occurring in the absence of an outside stimulus (e.g. hearing a voice outside one). Hallucinations are particularly common in schizophrenia. Patients hear voices which tell them to do things, comment on their actions, utter obscenities or murmur wordlessly. The phenomenon of 'hearing one's thoughts spoken aloud' is encountered in schizophrenia. Hallucinations are described as hypnagogic if they are experienced whilst falling asleep and hypnopompic if experienced whilst waking up.

Hypochondriasis

Preoccupation with fancied illness. Hypochondriacal features are common in depression and may be found as bizarre phenomena in schizophrenia. Hypochondriasis may be the central feature of a hysterical illness. It seems likely that hypochondriasis does not exist on its own but is usually a manifestation of some underlying psychiatric condition or personality disorder.

Illusion

A perceptual error or misinterpretation. These commonly occur in organic mental states, particularly delirium. A patient in such a state misinterpreted a building outside his window as being a liner about to sail.

Ideas of reference

The patient who has ideas of reference experiences events and perceives objects in his environment as having a special significance for himself. For example, a patient noticed that all the TV programmes she saw indicated to her in some unusual way that she had been singled out for observation by a secret police force.

Neurosis and psychosis

Although widely used the terms lack precise definition and give rise to disagreement. A working definition would be that neurotic illnesses are states in which anxiety, mild mood change and preservation of contact with reality are the rule. The neurotic patient is only too aware of his illness, and never loses contact with reality. In psychotic states the patient loses contact with reality, there is a tendency towards the more bizarre manifestations of psychiatric disturbance as a common finding. Mood change when present is likely to be profound. The neurotic has insight, the psychotic does not.

Thus it appears that we base our definitions of neurosis and psychosis on severity of symptoms rather than by anything else. Such an unsatisfactory state of affairs must persist until more is known about the aetiology of psychiatric disorders in general.

Mannerism

A habitual expressive movement of the face or body. Normal mannerisms are appropriate but pathological mannerisms are inappropriate (e.g. in schizophrenia).

Obsessional phenomena (obsessive compulsive phenomena)

These are contents of consciousness of an unpleasant and recurrent sort which the patient experiences as his or her own but which he or she resists. These contents may include words, ideas, phrases and acts. This is well exemplified by a patient who had to perform every act of washing, dressing and eating nine times or else he became anxious and distressed.

Paranoid

This is a widely known psychiatric term and about as widely misused. It derives from the Greek para noos, i.e. beyond reason. It has been used for years to describe 'classic' signs of psychosis—particularly those that encompass delusions of grandeur or those of a fantastic sort.

Recent use of the term has tended to assign to it the meaning of 'persecutory', thus paranoid delusions become delusions of persecution and suspicion, oversensitive people are regarded as 'paranoid'. This is no doubt related to the fact that ideas of persecution are commonplace in psychosis so that by a process of condensation paranoid = psychotic = persecuted. But this is an incorrect way of using the term which should be reserved for the formal description of delusions and syndromes characterized by 'persecution, grandeur, litigation, jealousy, love, envy, hate, honour, or the supernatural' (Lewis, 1970).

The term may be extended to describe the mechanism of projection by which a person refers events, even trifles, to himself, but it should be emphasized that the term implies a mechanism of psychotic intensity and not the sensitive ideas and feelings which are part of the normal experience of many.

Passivity feeling

A feeling of bodily influence or control by outside agents. This phenomenon is commonly found in schizophrenia.

Schizophrenia

A syndrome, occurring mainly in young people, in which are found character-istic disturbances of *thinking, perception, emotion* and *behaviour*. The illness tends to lead to disintegration of the personality.

Schizophrenic thought disorder

A characteristic type of disturbance of thinking, found only in schizophrenia, in which there is a basic disturbance of the process of conceptual thinking. This shows itself in the patient's speech, which reflects impaired logical thinking. Early schizophrenic thought disorder often manifests itself as a subjective difficulty in thinking clearly. In its most severe form thought disorder reduces patients' talk to fragmented nonsense—'word salad'. Certain German psychi-atrists have stressed the clinical importance of the patient's description of the feeling that thoughts are inserted into the head, or that they are being withdrawn from the head, or that one's thoughts are being spoken aloud outside of one *(Gedanken laut werden.)* Such manifestations are usually regarded as being of prime importance in making the diagnosis of schizophrenia.

General advice regarding the examination of and description of the mental state

The signs of mental disturbance can be elicited once the method is learned, in much the same way that one learns to elicit physical signs in general medicine. However, one should avoid leading questions, and it is also important to avoid making comments or remarks to the patient which may implant disruptive or disturbing ideas in his mind. In this way, one can avoid *interpreting* to the patient the *apparent meaning* of his experiences or feelings. Interpretation should be avoided and left to the expert. The patient should not be antagonized if he or she appears to be uncooperative. Antagonism, resistance and evasiveness can usually be overcome by handling the situation in a non-committal way. Recording the patient's talk verbatim is extremely useful, but may antagonize a prickly patient. A scheme for the mental state is given below.

Behaviour

In describing the patient's behaviour one should try as far as possible to get an accurate description of how the patient behaves during interview. One starts by observing the patient's behaviour, instead of just taking it for granted. Points to note include:

1   the patient's general level of consciousness;
2   awareness of what is going on around him or her;
3   level of cooperation with the examiner;
4   whether the patient is able to make contact with the examiner at interview;
5   predominant facial expressions and whether they are appropriate;
6   use of gesture;

7   activity—free or constrained, continuous or interrupted;
8   the presence of agitation; and
9   use of mannerisms.
This is not a complete list and is only intended as a guide.

Talk

It is usual to consider both the *form* and the *content* of the patient's talk. The form is the manner of talk, i.e. how it presents (sustained, interrupted, fast or slow, etc.). The simplest way to examine the content of the patient's talk is by making a verbatim sample. Content means the predominant topics.

Mood

Here we try to comment on whether the patient's mood is sustained or variable. What is the predominant mood as far as possible? Quite often a description of the patient's mood cannot be put down in one word, such as 'depressed'. A useful way of enquiring about the patient's mood is to ask some questions such as 'How do you feel in yourself?' or 'How are your spirits?'

Thought content

Delusions

These can only be elicited by careful questioning. Some patients will talk very spontaneously about their delusions and express a wide variety of illogical ideas. Other patients will need to be questioned. Paranoid delusions are often persecutory and to elicit them requires bland questions which do not arouse patients' suspicions too strongly. Such questions are 'Are people treating you as they should?' or 'How are people behaving towards you, do you suppose?' are often quite useful. Enquire about the patient's attitude to his or her own self. Ask whether the individual feels he or she has changed in any way, or considers him or herself to be a good or bad person. This may help to elicit feelings of guilt and self-recrimination.

Hypochondriacal ideas

It is important to recognize that hypochondriacal concern is an extremely common finding amongst psychiatric patients. Thus the anxious patient may have a considerable amount of hypochondriacal fear surrounding bodily symptoms of anxiety such as palpitations. On the other hand, the severely depressed patient may present with severe hypochondriasis which may well be missed by the examining doctor until he or she is aware of the significance of hypochondriasis in depression (q.v.). Bizarre hypochondriacal notions tend to be found in schizophrenic illnesses.

Obsessive compulsive phenomema

Here one should enquire about habits surrounding various aspects of the patient's daily life. For instance, the patient with an obsessional disorder may have rituals concerned with washing and eating, etc., which he or she feels obliged to carry out though they cause much discomfort. Very often the patient will be extremely ashamed of this type of symptom and discuss it only with difficulty. Compulsions are the motor concomitants of obsessions.

Perceptual disturbance

Here one records hallucinations and illusions, noting the modality of the hallucination and its content, and also the occasions on which they tend to occur.

Cognitive testing

Memory

The patient's account of his or her history when compared with other informants will give some assessment of his or her memory for past events. Recent memory may be adequately tested by asking the patient to give an acount of the preceding 24 hours. The ability to retain new information and reproduce it may be tested as follows:

1   Give the patient a name, address and telephone number. Ask him or her to repeat it immediately and to reproduce it in 5 minutes.

2   Ask the patient to listen to a sentence and repeat it exactly, e.g. 'One thing a nation must have to become rich and great is an adequate secure supply of wood.'

Orientation

Record the patient's account of the time of day, date and place. Also record who the patient thinks he or she is and who he or she thinks you are.

Concentration

One should record the patient's level of attention to the questions asked and also try and test concentrating ability by asking him or her to subtract 7 from 100 until he or she can go no further, noting the number of mistakes and the time taken.

General information and intelligence

Under the heading 'general information' one attempts to assess the individual's store of general knowledge. Useful questions here will include such things as the patient's familiarity with current affairs, topics of the day and familiarity with reigning figures and political names. Intelligence can be assessed quite roughly clinically bearing in mind the patient's educational background and professional attainments, and some attempt should be made to place a patient on the scale:

1   below average;

2   average;

3   above average.

Insight

Assessing patients' insight is the most difficult thing of all. It does not merely mean asking patients whether they know whether they are ill or not, although of course awareness of the existence of illness is an important criterion of insight. But in deciding and commenting upon the pateint's level of insight, one wants to know, too, how aware the patient is of the extent of his or her illness and its effect on other people, such as family, employers and colleagues. One wants to know too, whether the patient has any idea of how his or her illness seems to others or how he or she might feel about a similar illness in other people. Some idea about the patient's insight might be gleaned from his or her views regarding future plans, etc.

Special investigations

Special investigations of the mental state include the use of tests of psychological function. It is important to point out that there is no 'ideal' psychological test—a fact which surprises some students whose notions of clinical psychology are likely to be hazy. This is a professional discipline devoted to psychological investigation and, properly used, can clarify problems in diagnosis and guide, assess and plan treatment and rehabilitation. The sophisticated use of psychometry relies on the use of batteries of tests and careful selection of testing procedures by the psychologist and *not* by the doctor. Just as the physiologist is the scientific back-up to the physician, so the psychologist is to the psychiatrist.

Common areas of psychiatric scrutiny include the measurement of intelligence and assessment of personality structure.

Frequently used intelligence tests include the Raven Progressive Matrices and the Mill Hill Vocabulary Scale. These tests of general and verbal ability are well standardized, relatively simple to administer either to individuals or to groups, and give an acceptable assessment of the intelligence level. The Wechsler Adult Intelligence Scale (WAIS) is another well-standardized intelligence test which is more comprehensive than the former. It includes tests of performance as well as verbal tests.

Personality assessment relies first of all on questionnaires which are designed to identify patterns of personality structure. An example of this is the Minnesota Multiphasic Personality Inventory (MMPI). This questionnaire consists of over 500 items. The questions are designed to tap attitudes in the respondent which may be construed as indicating the presence of elements going to make up a particular personality structure, and also to reveal the presence of elements resembling at least certain clinical psychiatric syndromes. A more sophisticated test is the Millon Clinical Multiaxial Inventory (MCMI), which measures many psychological dimensions.

A psychological dimension is a continuum along which people may vary. For example, people are more or less intelligent, and more or less shy. Both of these are examples of familiar psychological dimensions. However, dimensions can be constructed by arbitrary questionnaires, their justification being that they correlate with something clinically useful. A good example of this is Rotter's 'locus of control' dimension which sees people as more or less externally or internally driven. The internally driven individual knows what he or she wants out of life, can generate his or her own purposes and usually pursue them with application. The externally driven has a locus of control outside him or herself and responds to events as a ball of paper in the street responds to the wind. For such individuals, life is a capricious series of random events.

Some investigators elevate a few dimensions to a significant assessment of personality. Eysenck's extraversion and neuroticism dimensions are an example.

Rating scales are used in research and mental state examination. Examples are the Hamilton rating scale for depression, scoring various symptoms and signs, and Goldberg's General Health Questionnaire (GHQ), especially used in general practice.

The suspicion that psychometry is dogged by subjective reflection on the part of the patient is hard to dispel. The noumenal matrices ('construct grids') of Kelly aim to avoid this by asking the subject to create his or her own significant variables and objectively assessing what that individual perceives as significant. These grids of belief are an interesting development, but so far psychologists have found difficulty harnessing them for clinical purposes.

Laboratory investigations

There are no routine investigations in psychiatric practice, although chest X-ray, skull X-ray and syphilitic serology still remain important investigations that every patient should have as well as a complete blood picture and urine analysis.

The advent of *computerized tomography* has made available one of the most revolutionary investigations in the exclusion of organic brain disease. Although no one would regard this as a routine investigation in psychiatric practice, it is beyond question that it will become frequently used in this field. Position emission tomograms ('PET scans') are a refinement. An electroence-phalogram (EEG) is usually confirmatory. Magnetic resonance imaging is also a most helpful method of investigation. A good rule is that the doctor should always have some good reason for using a special investigation rather than resorting to whole batteries of special tests.

Finally, the essentials of this history and mental state should be summarized in a formulation of the patient's illness, presenting a bird's eye view of the diagnosis, likely treatment and possible prognosis.

The proficient psychiatrist should be able to succinctly *formulate* a case in two or three sentences, e.g. 'This is a 44-year old carpenter with a 2-year history of obsessions and no previous illnesses. It followed his divorce and a previously regular methodical life. This is probably obsessional neurosis, but possibly depressive illness, which should respond to clomipramine.' The important features to elicit for a formulation are:

1   differential diagnosis;
2   identifiable precipitants; and
3   the pre-morbid personality.

Reference

Lewis, A. J. (1970) Paranoia and paranoid states: a historical perspective. *Psychological Medicine*, **1**, 2–12.

Further reading

Asch, S. (1988) *Social Psychology*. Oxford University Press, Oxford.

Bebbington, P. E. & Hill, P. D. (1985) *A Manual of Practical Psychiatry*. Blackwell Scientific Publications, Oxford.

Davis, D. R. (1984) *An Introduction to Psychopathology*. Oxford University Press, Oxford.

Fish, F. J. (1985) *Clinical Psychopathology*. John Wright, Bristol.

Fransella, F. (1976) Personal constructs. *Recent Advances in Clinical Psychiatry*, **2**, 81.

Freud, S. (1989) *Psychopathology of Everyday Life*. Penguin, London.

Jaspers, K. (1968) *General Psychopathology*. Manchester University Press, Manchester.

Kendell, R. (1975) *The Role of Diagnosis in Psychiatry*. Blackwell Scientific Publications, Oxford.

Schneider, K. (1959) *Clinical Psychopathology*. Grune & Straiton, London.

Shepherd, M. & Zangwill, O. L. (1983) *General Psychopathology*. Cambridge University Press, Cambridge.

Trimble, M. (1985) New brain imaging techniques and psychiatry. *Recent Advances in Clinical Psychiatry*, **5**, 225–44.

World Health Organisation (1988) ICD-IQ, Geneva.

Chapter 2
Affective Disorders

Introduction

The affective disorders are all characterized by a primary disturbance of mood, the polar extremes of which range from profound sadness and dejection in severe depression to the breezy, insightless hilarity of mania. Less severe varieties of mood disturbance may be seen in so-called neurotic depression and lead to a surprising degree of handicap. The common thread that unites all these disorders is mood disturbance, which is only recognized as a manifestation of illness when it is excessive and goes beyond the customary fluctuations of mood that are part of the fabric of ordinary mental life. In affective disorder, however, mood disturbance is not merely extreme, it is also disproportionate. Another important aspect of pathological mood change is that it is unresponsive to outside influence—the depressed patient is not easily reassured nor cheered up any more than is the hypomanic patient even slightly put off by comments on his or her exuberant behaviour. Any other manifestations occurring in affective disorder, whether they be physiologic or perceptual, are secondary and follow in the wake of the primary mood change.

Classification of affective disorders

Kräpelin was the first to describe manic depressive insanity, a disorder in which excitement and depression alternated. After Kräpelin, physicians looked beyond manic depressive disorders and became more aware of depression as a disorder on its own.

Depressions are often described either as being *reactive* or *endogenous*. Since these terms are in such common use some explanation must be made of them, but it is a fact that their use is controversial.

Reactive depression is usually so named if the depression can be shown to satisfy the following conditions: (i) Its onset follows some obvious cause in the patient's life, such as loss of a job, broken engagement, examination failure, etc; (ii) The content of the illness is concerned with the cause to the exclusion of everything else; (iii) the illness would not have come on if the precipitating event had not occurred. Many people prefer to use the term neurotic depression rather than reactive depression.

Endogenous depression is so named if: (i) The depression arises out of the blue, unrelated to external events; (ii) there is diurnal variation of mood; (iii) there is sleep disturbance with early morning wakening.

In practice the distinction between these two 'types' of depression is hard to make—what at first sight appears to be 'reactive' depression then turns out to be 'endogenous' by virtue of the presence of diurnal mood variation, early wakening, etc.

Current practice in the classification of depressions still reflects a division of opinion. In addition to the reactive (neurotic)–endogenous dichotomy of depression, other people have preferred to classify depressions as primary or secondary. A primary depressive state is one which arises apparently spontaneously and is not related to any preceding physical or psychiatric illness or unfavourable event.

Finally, it is now recognized that there are differences between these two types of severe affective disorder. Manic depressive illness or bipolar affective disorder is distinguished from unipolar disorder, which is always depressive in type and shows a different genetic inheritance, response to treatment and possibly a different biological basis.

Depression

In depression the mood resembles sadness or grief but is sustained, unlike the transitory mood changes that many people experience in response to various stresses or from one part of the day to the other. The important thing about depressive states is that this change of mood is sustained and that it exceeds these ordinary variations quantitatively and qualitatively. In addition, there are other bodily and emotional disturbances. There is no point in expanding the concept of depression in an attempt to explain away every variety of human unhappiness.

It is often hard to distinguish 'true' depression from states of unhappy malaise that trouble people with abnormal personalities, those who abuse drugs or alcohol or, for that matter, people with chronic painful illnesses. These are more than unhappiness, yet they are not depression—often they are referred to as states of 'dysphoria'. The accompaniments of depression are:

1 insomnia;
2 loss of energy;
3 loss of interest;
4 anorexia;
5 weight loss; and
6 decreased libido and impotence.

Aetiology

Incidence and prevalence

Depression is a common disorder. General practice consultation rates have been calculated at 31 per 1000 for neurotic depression—population surveys suggest even higher rates up to 15%.

Bipolar affective disorder and mania are rarer disorders with incidence rates of 0.6 and 0.02% in the general population respectively.

Heredity

Early attempts at identifying a genetic factor looked for genetic differences between endogenous and neurotic depression, but so much overlap was found as to render this idea untenable. Leonhard (1979) pointed out that a better dichotomy might be provided by separating affective disorders into bipolar (manic depressive) and unipolar (pure depression).

In general, the findings have been that unipolar psychoses and bipolar psychoses appear to breed true with very little overlap. The percentages of affected family members vary. Angst (1966) found the percentage of affected family members in bipolar psychosis to be 14.4% (parents) and 21.5% (sibs), and in unipolar psychosis 11.2% (parents) and 12.2% (sibs). Studies of twins suggest a concordance rate of around 70% in monozygotic and 19% in dizygotic twins of the same sex.

This strongly suggests a genetic influence in bipolar and unipolar psychoses which have been shown to breed true and which are relatively easy to identify. The mode of inheritance is not known. The majority view at present is that it is probably a polygenic type of inheritance. There is no evidence of genetic factors operating in neurotic depression.

Sex

In Western culture women are more frequently affected than men, with a ratio of 2 : 1.

Social class

Hitherto it was held that affective disorders are more common in social classes I and II of the population, in contrast to schizophrenia, which is more common in social classes IV and V; it should be remembered that more subtle social factors may operate at least to some extent. In the 'upper' social classes depression may be more likely to be recognized by patient and doctor. That this can be the case in America, at any rate, was shown by Hollingshead & Redlich (1958) who demonstrated that diagnosis and treatment were materially affected by membership of a particular social class. Upper class people were found to be more frequently diagnosed as neurotic and receive psychotherapy, while lower class people were more likely to be diagnosed as psychotic and receive electroconvulsive therapy (ECT), and these biases appeared to be determined by social class. More recent population studies in the UK have indicated an increased incidence in working class females, particularly those with two or more children. An incidence as high as 15–20% of the population studied was recorded.

Current findings favour a significantly higher incidence of depressive states in lower socioeconomic groups no matter how they are defined.

Constitution

1 *Body type.* The body type is more predominantly 'pyknic', i.e. small extremities and large visceral cavities (Mr Pickwick).

2 *Personality.* A personality type notable for swings of mood—'cyclothymic' personality—is a common accompaniment of affective disorder.

Many patients who develop mania have a pre-morbid personality notable for unusual jollity and energy—the so-called hypomanic personality.

Stress

The relationship of depression to apparent external causes is often obscure and misleading—causes invoked by patient or relative may be no more than an expression of the illness itself. For example, a man presented with a history of depression after dismissal from his job. On closer questioning it became clear that his symptoms of depression had antedated his sacking and that he had lost his job because of his incompetence, itself a manifestation of depression.

Age

Age plays a part in the aetiology of depression, some age groups being particularly vulnerable. Old age with loneliness and the fear of death is the most obvious example. Middle age can be particularly threatening, particularly for the striving man who suddenly arrives at this age and realizes he has accomplished less than he had hoped. If this coincides with the loss of his children by marriage, for example, it is liable to be all the harder to bear and frank depression may develop. Adolescence is a time of turmoil, and depression at this age, though rare, is severe when it does occur. The most severe depressions occur after the age of 60.

Physiological events precipitating depression

1   *Childbirth*, an event of physiological and psychological significance, is the first and most obvious example. Lability of mood is normal in the puerperium, but acute severe depression does occur and needs prompt recognition and treatment.
2   *The menopause* is a time of hormonal and psychological change and is often accompanied by depression.
3   *Acute febrile illnesses*, such as influenza, can trigger off depression.
4   *Chronic illness*, particularly chronic painful illness, is commonly accompanied by depression. Unfortunately this depression often passes unrecognized since it can be relieved and the illness made more easy to bear.
5   *Jaundice*.

Social factors

Social isolation and insecurity with loneliness and accompanying despair probably account for a large proportion of chronic depression.

Drugs

Many drugs can cause depression, including the sulphonamides, methyl dopa, reserpine, phenobarbitone and any of the contraceptive pills, particularly those with a high progesterone content. Steroids can cause depression—usually during withdrawal, and depressive states are common in withdrawal from amphetamines. Also, certain antiparkinsonian drugs, such as benzhexol, may cause depression or even states of excitement and confusion. Many antihypertensives have depressant effects or interfere with antidepressant chemotherapy.

Clinical manifestations

Mood change

Mood change is fundamental in *every* depressive illness. Here it is worth noting that one should not confuse the lay and medical usage of the term 'depression'. When we talk of depression we refer to a clinical entity, formerly distinguished by the word 'melancholia' (from the Greek, *melagkholia*: (too much) black bile), and do not use it loosely to describe transitory feelings of sadness or dejection.

The depressed patient's mood colours his or her entire mental life; thus in severe depression an individual will form incorrect judgements—delusional ideas based on altered mood, e.g. a patient may say that he has been condemned to death for his numerous misdeeds.

Such severe depression is uncommon; much more common is a general depressive colouring to the patient's outlook. The world seems grey and dark, the future appears grim and the patient sees him or herself as a failure unworthy of anyone's pity or affection. People who feel like this are likely to attempt suicide. Ideas of guilt and unworthiness are extremely common in depression.

Psychomotor activity

Alteration in psychomotor activity follows in the wake of mood change. The patient's movements and talk are slow and ponderous. This is called retardation. The patient is aware of this and often describes slowness in thought and difficulty in concentration. These latter can be elicited by simple tests of concentration, such as the serial subtraction of 7 from 100.

Poor concentration shows itself in the patient's work or studies and is confirmed by colleagues who comment that he or she is not coping with work as well as formerly. The housewife finds that work piles up in the home whilst she sits around in a hopeless state unable to concentrate but feeling sad and dejected. Frank weeping is not particularly common in depression. Far more common is the statement 'I've got past the stage of being able to cry. I can't cry any more. Perhaps I'd feel better if I could.'

Sleep disturbance

Insomnia is very common in depression and may be manifest as delayed sleep, broken sleep or early waking. Early waking is said to be the most common form of persistent sleep disorder. The patient wakes in the early hours and is unable to sleep, thereafter he or she remains awake for a few hours before getting up unrefreshed. Often bad dreams occur.

Other bodily disturbances

By day the patient lacks energy, interest and appetite. Weight loss is common. Apathy and loss of interest may be the presenting symptoms of depression. Hypochondriacal concern is commonly found, particularly centring on the bowels, which are often constipated.

Other psychological accompaniments

Anxiety is encountered in almost *every* depressive illness—there is no point in attempting clinical separation of anxiety from depression. Elderly depressed patients usually show agitation, that is to say restless, semi-purposive overactivity with hand wringing and inability to sit or lie still. Agitation can sometimes be so severe as to resemble manic excitement, except that the affect is one of hopelessness and despair. Paranoid features, particularly in middle-aged and elderly patients, may dominate the clinical picture in depression.

Hysterical symptoms can either mask depression or complicate the picture. In the first instance failure to recognize the essential depressive nature of the illness can be very dangerous, particularly when the hysterical symptom is protecting the patient from a suicidal impulse.

Hypochondriasis is extremely common in depressive states—in its most severe form one finds hypochondriacal delusions in the severely depressed patient. More common, perhaps, is the finding of a pervasive hypochondriacal attitude in the concern about the bodily accompaniments of depression, such as constipation. Very often this hypochondriasis is the presenting symptom of depression and may bring the patient initially to the attention of an investigating physician rather than a psychiatrist.

In summary, it can be said that current views on the symptomatology of major depressive illness in those that some would describe as endogenous, psychotic or primary are:

1   an autonomous cause;
2   a need for biological treatment; and
3   a presumed alteration in brain biochemistry.

There is now solid evidence to suggest that the primary and most important symptoms in these major depressive states are psychomotor retardation, agitation, feelings of self blame and decreased concentration in addition to mood change.

Differential diagnosis

Important physical disorders to be excluded are:

1   *Myxoedema.* Remembering that in myxoedema, depression and paranoid psychoses are commonly manifestations of the underlying disorder.
2   *Parkinsonism.* Depression is a common accompaniment of parkinsonism.
3   *Myasthenia gravis.*
4   *Addison's disease.*

The important psychiatric conditions to be distinguished from depression are:

1   *Schizophrenia.* Though the presence of thought disorder and true delusions may make the diagnosis of schizophrenia on occasions comparatively simple, it has to be remembered that the prodrome of schizophrenia may be apparently entirely depressive, hence adolescent depression should be diagnosed very cautiously.
2   *Dementia.* Presence of signs of organic deterioration should make diagnosis of dementia possible, though atypical depressions may simulate dementia and depression may complicate the disorder.

Complications of depression

1   *Suicide and attempted suicide.* All depressed patients should be carefully assessed for the possibility of suicide. Threats should never be ignored and must always be carefully evaluated. It is very important always to remember that there are a number of rather foolish statements about suicide which must be disregarded. First of these is 'a patient who talks about suicide won't do it'; nothing could be further from the truth. There are some generally agreed pointers which may indicate an impending suicidal attempt, and they include severe sleep disturbance with increased concern about it; a history of previous suicidal attempt; a family history of suicide; suicidal talk and preoccupation; severe hypochondriasis; associated physical illness; social isolation; and persistent feelings of guilt and self-depreciation.

In recent years the taking of tablets in the form of deliberate overdose has become so common in hospital practice that some have suggested that the term attempted suicide for these people should be discarded and that this should be referred to as self-poisoning. At all events, whatever the condition is called, it should always be remembered that from time to time people will take drugs such as sleeping pills in doses in excess of therapeutic level in an attempt to blot out reality by deep sleep and also as a way of drawing attention to their personal or social problems. This is not to suggest that all suicidal attempts constitute a serious psychiatric emergency, but rather that every one of these attempts should be evaluated by the physician with careful regard to the individual's personal and social situation.

2   *Malnutrition.*

3   *Worsening of coexisting physical disease.* This may occur through neglect, etc., pulmonary tuberculosis or diabetes mellitus.

4   *Abuse of drugs or alcohol.* This may happen in an attempt to 'fight off' depression.

Treatment

Of all psychiatric disorders depression is the most treatable. Nowadays the majority of depressives are treated as outpatients, but admission to hospital will always be necessary for severe depression, particularly where there is suicidal risk.

General measures

In the present era of physical treatments, the possibility of spontaneous remission is not awaited since most psychiatrists rightly feel that the patient's suffering should not be needlessly prolonged. It should be remembered, however, that good psychiatric nursing and sedation will always provide comfort and some degree of improvement to the depressed patient.

Physical treatment

1   *Electroconvulsive therapy (ECT).* ECT is widely regarded as a very useful antidepressant treatment in severe depressive states, but with the advent of the antidepressant drugs its usage has declined. Also, many psychiatrists are beginning to seriously question the value of ECT (see Chapter 13).

2 *Antidepressant drugs.* The antidepressant drugs include the tricyclic antidepressants and the monoamine oxidase inhibitors. Some of these medications are discussed more fully in Chapter 13. In general the tricyclic drugs are much more widely used than the monoamine oxidase inhibitors which have serious disadvantages from the point of view of side-effects, and it appears that the latter type of drug has a much less definite place in the treatment of depression. It should be added that at the present time too, the place of tricyclic antidepressants is being questioned by many since it is possible that they are excessively used. Nevertheless, the antidepressant drugs remain the mainstay of the treatment of depression.

3 *Psychotherapy.* Usually supportive.
4 *Occupational therapy.*
5 *Social rehabilitation.*
6 *Cognitive therapy* (*see* Chapter 13).

Prognosis

Depression tends to recur. It may well be that prolonged medication with antidepressant drugs helps to avert recurrence, though it is too early to be definite about this. The average duration of hospitalization in depression is about 6 weeks.

Mania

Mania is less common than depression and tends to be an acute and more circumscribed illness. Chronic depression is commonplace—chronic mania does not exist. *Hypomania* is the term used to describe mild or moderate degrees of mania.

Aetiology

1 See 'Depression'.
2 *Pre-morbid personality.* Commonly the manic patient is found to have either a cyclothymic personality or else to have always been more energetic and cheerful than his or her fellows (hypomanic personality).

Clinical manifestations

Mood

The mood is one of cheerfulness—or hilarity. Manic patients are described as showing infectious jollity—soon everyone in the room is laughing with them. This is often true, but the jollity is more often than not laced with irritability and flashes of anger, particularly if someone disagrees with them. Manic patients deny all symptoms and say they have never felt better in their lives. They are optimistic and have elaborate plans for the future, not only their own futures but for anyone else who cares to take advantage of the plans they are making. The plans at first may be sensible, if a little overenthusiastically stated, but sooner or later they become grandiose as such patients' critical sense fades. The manic patient's insight about his or her lack of judgement is practically nil in mania.

Sudden mood changes with transient bouts of tearful sadness are also encountered.

Activity
The overactivity in mania follows naturally from the feeling of general well-being that patients experience. Their energy is boundless. They get up before everyone else in the house and go to bed long after exhausted members of the family have retired. At work they go from one project to another, completing nothing. They overspend, buy all sorts of things, dress extravagantly and invite large numbers of unexpected friends home. As activity increases, so the patients' attention decreases so that they are increasingly unable to concentrate on anything.

Talk
Talk reflects the cheery mood and increased activity. The stream of talk gradually increases until it becomes torrential. It flits from topic to topic (flight of ideas) and associations are casual, often triggered by rhymes or puns. Jokes are frequent.

Delusions
True delusions are not found but manic patients do form delusional ideas based on their overoptimistic views of life in general. It is also not uncommon to find the irritable manic showing a paranoid attitude, particularly when objections are made to his or her plans.

Bodily disturbance
1 Sleep is lost through excessive energy.
2 Appetite is often voracious without any weight gain.
3 Libido is heightened.
4 Abuse of alcohol is common.

Mode of onset
Onset is usually acute and the duration of a manic illness is on the average about 6–8 weeks.

Hypomania often passes unrecognized at first, it is merely remarked by relatives that the patient had seemed full of zest and cheeriness for a few weeks and then things seemed to get out of hand.

Some manic illnesses terminate abruptly, others swing into depression.

Differential diagnosis
1 *Schizophrenias.* The presence of true thought disorder and delusions should make simple the diagnosis of these from mania. In practice it is often difficult to be precise about states of excitement. Time usually clarifies the picture. Mania occurs episodically, usually with intervals of complete recovery. This is rarely the case with schizophrenia.
2 *Drug-induced excitment*, e.g. amphetamine and its derivatives.

Treatment

    1 *Admission to hospital.*

    2 *Attention to feeding.* Manic patients may be so overactive that they stop eating for a few days before admission. This means that they arrive in hospital exhausted and dehydrated. As a consequence their mental state may be the more disturbed through vitamin depletion.

    3 *Medication.*

        (a) Sedatives. Immediate sedation to calm a wildly excited patient can be used, but this has generally been replaced by the use of neuroleptics.

        (b) Neurolpetics. Neuroleptic drugs are extremely useful in calming manic excitement and those most commonly used include: (i) chlorpromazine—up to 1 g per 24 hours in divided doses; (ii) thioridazine (Melleril); (iii) haloperidol— the starting dose of haloperidol given to an excited patient may be 5 mg intramuscularly and, thereafter, the dose repeated every hour until the patient has calmed down. After this the patient can usually be managed on much smaller doses by mouth.

    4 *ECT.* ECT has a definite place in the treatment of mania. It is usually given with neuroleptics.

    5 *Lithium.* Lithium was first recognized as a psychotropic drug as long ago as 1897, had a bad reputation for toxicity until 1949 when interest in its use was revived. Present uses are:

    (a) treatment of acute manic states;

    (b) treatment of recurrent manic states; and

    (c) treatment of chronic depressive states.

    In the case of acute mania it appears to have a definite place, though its value in recurrent mania, i.e. as a prophylactic drug, is less certain. Its place in the treatment of chronic depression is very uncertain. The drug is given as lithium carbonate, usually at a dose of 200–600 mg tds, levelling off to a lower maintenance dose. Its toxic effects necessitate frequent monitoring of the serum lithium level which should not rise above 0.5–1.5 mEq/l. Toxic effects include the following:

    (a) Gastrointestinal effects—anorexia, nausea, vomiting and diarrhoea.

    (b) Neuromuscular effects—weakness, tremor, ataxia and choreo-athetosis.

    (c) CNS effects—incontinence, dysarthria, blurred vision, dizziness, fits, retardation, somnolence and confusion, stupor, coma.

    (d) Cardiovascular effects—pulse irregularities, ECG changes, circulatory collapse. Other effects: polyuria, polydipsia, dehydration.

    Because of its toxicity, lithium should not be given to anyone with any degree of renal impairment. In general it is a drug that should only be used in the setting of inpatient and outpatient hospital care.

Conclusion

    In general, of the affective disorders it can be said that depression is a particularly common disorder, amenable to treatment by a wide variety of methods, but one which can cause a great deal of hardship. For this reason it should not pass unrecognized. In the treatment of depression a good rule to abide by is that if the patient is not showing signs of improvement with a particular line of treatment, this line of treatment should not be pushed to the level of absurdity before trying something else.

References

Angst, J. (1966) *Zur Aetiologie und Nosologie endogener depressiver Psychosen.* Springer, Berlin.

Hollingshead, A.B. & Redlich, F.C. (1958) *Social Class and Mental Illness: a Community Study.* Wiley, New York.

Further reading

Färgemann, P. M. (1963) *Psychogenic Psychoses.* Butterworths, London.

Kendell, R. E. (1976) The classification of depressions. *British Journal of Psychiatry,* **139**, 15.

Kleist, K. (1974) The cycloid psychoses. In Hirsch, S. R. & Shepherd, M. (Eds) *Themes and Variations in European Psychiatry.* John Wright. Bristol.

Kräpelin, E. (1921) *Manic Depressive Insanity and Paranoia.* Churchill Livingstone, Edinburgh.

Leonhard, K. (1979) *The Classification of Endogenous Psychoses.* Irvington, New York.

Nelson J. C. & Charney, D. S. (1981) The symptoms of major depressive illness: criteria for melancholia. *Archives of General Psychiatry,* **38**, 555–9.

Perris, C. (1974) *Cycloid Psychoses.* Munksgaard, Copenhagen. (*Acta Psychiatrica Scandinavica,* Supplement 253.)

Chapter 3
Schizophrenia

Definition

Schizophrenia is a syndrome in which are found specific, clinically recognizable psychological manifestations, occurring before age 45 and commonly leading to disintegration of the personality. Schizophrenics have peculiar ways of thinking and behaving and perceive their environment in an abnormal way. They have an inner life dominated by fantastic ideas, their emotional display is incongruous and they are cut off from their fellows so that they appear to have withdrawn from the world. The syndrome was originally described by Kräpelin (1913) who delineated its essentials under the name 'dementia praecox'. This was a fundamental step in the history of descriptive psychiatry since up till that time what we now recognize as schizophrenia was buried in a multitude of apparently dissimilar syndromes. The name 'schizophrenia' was applied by Bleuler who viewed the syndrome as being based on a process of psychological disintegration manifesting itself ultimately as a fragmentation of the personality. He also considered it a group of similar syndromes, 'the schizophrenias' with a variety of aetiology (Bleuler 1950).

Aetiology

Incidence

The incidence of schizophrenia is found to be 0.85% of the general population. This figure is remarkably constant, whatever populations are surveyed.

Heredity

The precise role of heredity in schizophrenia is uncertain and the means of inheritance is unknown. It is possible to calculate the expectancy of schizophrenia in the family of the schizophrenic, where the incidence in the proband's parents may be between 5% and 10% and in full sibs between 5% and 15% (see also Table 1). Twin studies used to be quoted as showing a concordance rate of up to 80% in monozygotic twins but the figure is now said to be 60%, though some put it as low as 30%. Schizophrenia breeds true in families (Table 1); on the other hand 60% of schizophrenics have no family history of the syndrome. Although genetics are obviously important, they clearly only account for half the variance in the case of monozygotic twins.

Personality

Many writers have stressed the importance of the pre-morbid personality structure of the schizophrenic. As ever one is confronted with the difficulty of assessing personality, but even so a 'schizoid personality' has been described. This is a personality type which appears to contain the seeds of schizophrenia.

Table 1 Approximate guide to likelihood of schizophrenia in relatives of a sufferer

Relationship to patient	Chance of schizophrenia (%)
None	1
Second degree relative (e.g. aunt, nephew)	2
Child	5
Parent	7
Sibling	10
Monozygotic twin	50

Schizoid individuals display behavioural traits such as seclusiveness, abnormal shyness, hypochondriasis, emotional coolness and indifference, fanaticism and eccentricity. However, various workers have found some difference in the incidence of these abnormal personalities before the onset of schizophrenia. Bleuler (1950) found a 34% incidence of schizoid personality in a series of schizophrenics. Other workers have found a higher incidence but it has to be admitted that up to 50% of schizophrenics show no evidence of previous personality disorder. Nevertheless the findings of personality disorder in an individual suspected of the slow development of schizophrenia may be a useful pointer towards the diagnosis. Further evidence of the role played by personality abnormality in the aetiology of schizophrenia is demonstrated by the increased incidence of deviant individuals in the families of schizophrenics.

Body build

The incidence of the asthenic body structure has been commented on by many workers. This type of body build is of poor prognostic significance, tending to be associated with chronicity.

Family experience

Much has been written concerning ambiguous management in the upbringing of children, but it is mostly speculative and often ends in unfortunate blaming of parents who are suffering enough already. Leff & Vaughn (1981) have shown the potency of certain family dynamics in provoking relapse in schizophrenia. They measured a variable called 'expressed emotion' and showed that reducing the exposure of the patient to antagonistic exchanges with his family was as effective as phenothiazines in preventing relapse.

It is difficult to evaluate dynamic theories of schizophrenic aetiology but it should not be thought that their explanatory and speculative nature makes them in any way mutually exclusive compared with biological theories. Far from it, schizophrenia is a heterogeneous collection of syndromes and no unitary theory of causality is acceptable on the evidence presently available.

Biochemistry

There is a growing body of evidence to suggest that the disturbance of schizophrenia may be biochemically transmitted. It has to be conceded that to date no specific biochemical effect has been identified as having an exclusive association with schizophrenia. Production of the so-called 'model psychoses' in volunteers following the administration of lysergic acid diethylamide (LSD) and mescaline was probably the first step in the investigation of the biochemistry of schizophrenia. However, perhaps the foremost indication of a biochemical disturbance and a neuropathological disturbance in the aetiology of schizophrenia was provided first of all by recognition of psychoses triggered off by taking amphetamines and secondly by the investigation of psychoses associated with temporal lobe epilepsy. In both these conditions, psychoses are produced which are clinically indistinguishable from schizophrenia. It was the further investigation of the amphetamine-induced psychoses that has led to the *dopamine hypothesis*. In this, it is postulated that the symptoms of schizophrenia are related to a functional excess of structurally normal dopamine. Amphetamines induce dopamine overactivity while at the same time it is found that antipsychotic drugs reduce it, presumably by blocking dopamine receptors. Biochemical hypotheses of schizophrenia have included the transmethylation hypothesis in which it is proposed that schizophrenic symptoms are caused by the accumulation of an abnormal biogenic amine. Other lines of enquiry relate to the possibility that schizophrenia is in fact an encephalitis produced by a slow virus and in addition to this considerable interest has been raised by finding ventricular dilation in chronic schizophrenics indicating a degree of cerebral atrophy which could well be related to a slow virus disorder, or obstetric trauma.

Physical illness

Physical happenings such as illnesses, operations or accidents can commonly precipitate an acute schizophrenic psychosis or bring about a remission in an established one.

Life changes

Recent research suggests that schizophrenic onset and relapse are significantly preceded by life changes, such as moving house, loss of a job, bereavement, etc. The implication of this may be that the schizophrenic has a low tolerance for change or overstimulation.

Psychological factors

The role of psychological factors in the aetiology of schizophrenia is far from clear. Common clinical experience teaches us that the schizophrenic may have the illness triggered off by any variety of psychological stress. Some self-limiting acute episodes appear clearly related to psychological precipitants. Färgemann (1963) consequently called them 'psychogenic psychoses' and followed a cohort, contrasting their good prognosis to other schizophrenics.

A comprehensive theory of the aetiology of schizophrenia would postulate that the schizophrenic process is mediated biochemically, i.e. it follows a biochemical final common path, the illness occurs in a genetically predisposed individual and it may be triggered off by a variety of physical or psychological stresses or both. It would certainly seem at present that this theory of multiple aetiology would be the most profitable one to follow in research. Schizophrenia therefore appears to be a complex disturbance occurring at many levels in which hereditary, psychological, neurophysiological, sociological and biochemical factors may all play relevant parts.

Clinical manifestations

These are best considered under the following headings: schizophrenic thought disorder; delusions; emotional disturbance; perceptual disturbance; and behavioural disturbance.

The reason for commencing with thought disorder lies in the fact that Bleuler in his original description of schizophrenia stressed the central position of the disturbance of thinking found in schizophrenia.

Schizophrenic thought disorder

This is a characteristic disturbance of the thought process peculiar to the schizophrenic syndrome. Schizophrenics' powers of thinking are impaired, i.e. their *powers of conceptual thinking are altered*, so that they may interchange cause and effect and draw entirely illogical conclusions from false premises. This will manifest itself by the finding that their talk is difficult to follow. When one examines an example of this talk one finds that the patient has said much but got little across. Closer examination reveals he or she has uttered a stream of nonsense. Subjectively patients may be aware of impaired thinking ability and may tell an examiner that they find it hard to think clearly or that their thoughts are vague, they cannot concentrate or somehow their thoughts wander. It may be necessary to use leading questions to elicit this information from a patient. As thought disorder is manifest in language, it has been suggested that schizophrenics are forced to construct for themselves a private language to explain their illogical ideas to themselves and others.

Attention is often drawn to the phenomenon of *thought blocking*. Here the patient's stream of thought is interrupted and a new line of thinking begins. It is shown by gaps in the patient's talk and found too in states of exhaustion and depressive retardation. Thought blocking is therefore *not peculiar to schizophrenia*. All the foregoing comments on schizophrenic thought disorder presuppose that the individual is of adequate intelligence. The diagnosis of schizophrenic thought disorder in the presence of subnormal intelligence would be very difficult.

The schizophrenic may experience interruption of thinking and tell the examiner that *thoughts are being withdrawn* (thought withdrawal) from his or her head, or that thoughts are being inserted into his or her head. This sort of complaint is absolutely diagnostic of schizophrenia and occurs in no other condition. In addition, the schizophrenic may experience transmission of his or her own thoughts to others. The term 'schizophrenic thought disorder' refers to the *specific disturbance of conceptual thinking* mentioned at the beginning of this section.

Delusions

A delusion is defined as an incorrect belief which is inappropriate to the individual's sociocultural background, and which is held in the face of logical argument. True delusions are fundamental errors in judgment and are as inexplicable as they are incomprehensible. They appear suddenly and are held with particular conviction. A distinction is drawn between these true or primary delusions and delusional ideas, since primary delusions are completely incomprehensible whereas delusional ideas are false but nevertheless explicable in the light of the patient's altered emotional state. For instance, in severe depression an individual can develop delusional ideas which can be explained on the grounds of his or her being sad and therefore believing that his or her life is finished, the future is hopeless, etc. The delusion proper is unshakeable, incorrect and held without insight. The content of a patient's delusion reflects his or her past experience and is coloured by his or her culture pattern. Thus 100 years ago religious content in delusions was much more common than it is at the moment. Nowadays it is common for deluded patients to believe that they are being persecuted by political organizations such as the Fascists or Communists, or that they are being influenced by atomic explosions, radioactivity, radar, television, etc. A deluded patient may also experience *ideas of reference*. This is an experience in which the patient finds that mundane happenings of even the most trifling sort have special meaning and significance for, or are directed particularly towards him or her. Thus a patient finds references to herself in the personal column of *The Times*, or another patient turns on a TV programme and discovers that all the characters are making remarks about him. *Passivity feelings* are commonly found in schizophrenia. In this the individual feels that his or her body or mind are under the influence of or being controlled by other people. Though paranoid delusions are not always present in schizophrenic illness, a paranoid colouring is common.

Emotional disturbance

Affective incongruity is typically found in severe schizophrenic illnesses. In this the patient's emotional display is inappropriate to his or her condition. In its most crude form one finds a patient laughing callously when being given some tragic news, or when talking of some serious happening. In the majority of instances we find that the emotional incongruity of schizophrenia is not so marked as the lack of emotional rapport which one can make with a schizophrenic. Many people have spoken of the pane of glass which separates one from the schizophrenic patient. It is difficult to identify with or empathize with schizophrenics. Their emotional display is limited: they are cool, detached and rather 'couldn't care less'. They are unmoved by various things going on around them and concerned only with their own private world. Other variations of emotion are found in schizophrenia too. It is not uncommon for a schizophrenic illness to be ushered in by a state of depression or anxiety or even mild hypomanic excitement. In fact, it is fair to say that any adolescent patient who presents with severe anxiety, inexplicable depression or acute hypomanic excitement must be suspected of a developing schizophrenia until it has been proven otherwise.

Perceptual disturbance

The commonest perceptual disturbance of schizophrenia is the hallucination, which is most commonly auditory. It is important always to enquire closely into the content and nature of the hallucinations. Patients may hear voices commenting on their actions, speaking their own thoughts aloud, uttering obscene words or phrases or telling them what to do. The voices may be familiar or unfamiliar, single or multiple. The majority of schizophrenic patients develop hallucinations at one stage or another during the illness.

Behavioural disturbance

In the development of schizophrenia one looks for alteration of the total behaviour of the individual rather than isolated phenomena. Often the relatives will describe how the individual has become more and more reclusive over a period of months, has appeared odd and made use of unfamiliar gestures, and has shunned friends and familiar activities. States of ecstasy, wild excitement and impulsive behaviour also occur in schizophrenia but probably the most common finding is a general falling off in activity. The scholar becomes less studious and the professional person less interested in and less able to perform his or her work. Periods of apparent inactivity may be interspersed with occasional bouts of rather purposeless enthusiasm for some hobby or other. Thus a schizophrenic was said to be spending much time on 'research'. When investigated this turned out to be a method of preserving butterflies' wings in some plastic substance which was somehow allied to a thesis on biochemistry. Outbursts of violence or senseless criminal acts are fortunately rare but can occur. Altered moral standards may be seen in developing schizophrenia, thus a previously puritanical young girl may become promiscuous, and it may be this concern about her sexual morals which brings her parents to consult the doctor, and the diagnosis of schizophrenia made. Any history of personality change in a young person must always raise the suspicion of schizophrenia.

Clinical types

Nowadays less importance is attached to the naming of clinical types. The making of the diagnosis, indeed establishing the concept of schizophrenia, is often hard enough! The clinical types which are described include:

1 *Simple schizophrenia*. Characterized by a general lowering of all mental activity. The simple schizophrenic presents with poverty of activity, volition, affect and thought. This variety of schizophrenia is most commonly confused with mental subnormality. Indeed the two clinical pictures may be indistinguishable. The onset is usually slow and insidious and the prognosis in general very bad.

2 *Hebephrenia*. As its name implies this is seen in the younger age groups and typically the clinical picture is one of rather fatuous euphoria and hallucinosis. Here the onset tends to be insidious and the prognosis bad. Thought disorder is usually marked.

3 *Paranoid schizophrenia*. Characterized by the development of systems of paranoid delusions. The onset is slow and insidious. Paranoid schizophrenia is

often associated with considerable preservation of the personality, so that the paranoid schizophrenic may be able to remain for a considerable time in the community and conceal his paranoid delusions. It is found in older age groups (30 and over).

4 *Catatonic schizophrenia.* This refers to a type where disorder of motor activity—hyperactivity or episodes of immobility—are prominent. It is rarely seen since the advent of phenothiazines and those cases that are seen as often as not turn out to be severe manic depression or organic brain disease.

General comments on diagnosis

A central problem in the diagnosis of schizophrenia has been the poor level of agreement amongst psychiatrists about definition of the term. Essentially schizophrenia comprises:

1   certain psychotic features such as delusions, thought disorder, hallucinations and emotional blunting;

2   a deterioration in function;

3   onset before age 40; and

4   a duration measured in months rather than days.

The lack of agreement on definition has led to the development of ten different operational definitions, one of which, that of Feighner (Feighner *et al.*, 1972), is as follows. Three categories, of required symptoms, A–C, are given:

Feighner's definition of schizophrenia

A

1   A chronic illness with at least 6 months of symptoms without return to the pre-morbid level of adjustment; and

2   absence of a period of depressive or manic symptoms sufficient to qualify for actual or probable affective disorder.

B   At least one of:

1   delusions or hallucinations without significant perplexity or disorientation; or

2   verbal production that makes communication difficult because of lack of logical or understandable organization.

C   At least three of:

1   single state;

2   poor pre-morbid social adjustment or work history;

3   family history of schizophrenia;

4   absence of alcoholism or drug abuse within 1 year of onset of the psychosis; or

5   onset of illness prior to age 40.

If only two of the requirements in category C are present, the diagnosis is 'probably' schizophrenia.

On the other hand, Schneider (1974) stressed the importance of 'first rank symptoms', namely audible thoughts, voices heard arguing, voices commenting on one's actions, the experience of influences playing on the body (somatic passivity experiences), thought withdrawal and other interferences with thought; diffusion of thought, delusional perception and all feelings, impulses (drives) and volitional acts that are experienced by the patient as the work or influence of others.

Definition and diagnosis then, are far from satisfactory but they are improving. This author tends to the use of Schneider's criteria and observation of the evolution of the disorder. The development of the disorder is often the best pointer to the diagnosis.

Differential diagnosis

1 *Affective disorder.*
2 *Drug-induced psychosis,* e.g. amphetamines, LSD or other hallucinogenic drugs.
3 *Organic psychosis.* Here the presence of clouded consciousness will be the critical diagnostic point.
4 *Personality disorder.*
5 *Hysteria.*
6 *Paranoid states.* Not everyone who becomes paranoid is schizophrenic!
7 *Psychosis associated with epilepsy.*

Treatment

No psychiatric topic is more beset with pitfalls than the treatment of schizophrenia. Since the condition is poorly comprehended it is difficult to treat adequately and impossible to treat specifically. This leads on the one hand to therapeutic nihilism and neglect of the patient and on the other to overtreatment based on tenuous theory, making the syndrome a perpetual testing ground. It is difficult to know which is the more dangerous of the two alternatives.

The treatment of the schizophrenic patient should consist of a *total approach to the patient,* aiming at strengthening the patient's ties with reality and rehabilitating him or her. In the acute state of the illness the patient may need to be in hospital and may have to be protected from him or herself since suicide commonly occurs in schizophrenia—he or she may need to be calmed by sedatives and tranquillizers, and his or her general state of health may need investigation for coexisting physical diseases which, if found, are appropriately treated.

At present the phenothiazine drugs, particularly *chlorpromazine* and *trifluoperazine,* are found particularly useful for influencing the mental state of this schizophrenic. These drugs not only calm but also alter perception and modify thinking. Chlorpromazine is given orally (50–200 mg tds) or by injection. Trifluoperazine is given orally (5–15 mg tds). Intramuscular injection of fluphenazine (Modecate) 25 mg monthly or flupenthixol (Depixol) 20 mg monthly is now established as an effective medication which many now regard as the treatment of choice. Dystonic and other extrapyramidal reactions are common but usually respond well to antiparkinsonian drugs. Occasionally they can be severe, chronic and quite refractory to treatment. They are then called *tardive dyskinesias*. 'Drug holidays', when the intramuscular phenothiazine is discontinued, should be considered if tardive dyskinesia appears to be developing despite anticholinergics.

Psychotherapy plays a part in the treatment of schizophrenia. It is of a supportive and re-integrative rather than analytic type. A psychotic patient cannot tolerate interpretations of his or her behaviour, and indeed such therapy can often be dangerously disruptive.

It is important to find useful and variable occupation for the patient. This may start with traditional occupational therapy. On the other hand there is much evidence to suggest that occupation of a constructive sort may be particularly valuable. The current interest in the reclamation of the chronic schizophrenic has shown the value of 'industrial therapy'. In industrial therapy units, chronic schizophrenics perform meaningful tasks producing various objects, e.g. light industrial assembly work, emphasis being placed on making the situation as near to a normal work situation as possible. This encourages patients to adopt a normal working role, and prepares them for a return to the community and the consequent return to gainful occupation.

Community care

No schizophrenic patient can be adequately treated in a social vacuum. For this reason it is important for the doctor concerned to know as much as possible about the patient's family and home conditions. The patient who comes from a family in which there are close ties and supportive interest is liable to make better progress than the one who is socially isolated or where the family is antagonistic.

Community care should therefore be more comprehensive than hospital care and is based on outpatient clinics and day hospitals. The object of community care is to avoid hospital admission wherever possible in order to avert the institutionalized apathy that the schizophrenic can so readily develop. The Mental Health Act has invested the local authority with the responsibility of organizing such services and in certain areas they are highly developed. There is always the danger, however, that the patient may be overlooked if communication is poor and the general practitioner, the hospital doctors and the local authority each assume that he or she is being looked after by the other two. Well-organized community care involves highly developed social work by psychiatric social workers, community psychiatric nurses and others in collaboration with the hospital psychiatrists. Ideally the whole operation should be part of a comprehensive, community-orientated mental health service.

There is much more to the follow up of patients discharged from hospital than mere attendance at an outpatient clinic now and again to receive further medication. The family of the schizophrenic patient requires rather more than simple reassurance. The presence of a psychotic member in the family can be enormously disrupting and may evoke every sort of emotional response. To ignore this and discharge a patient to an unprepared family is to invite early readmission. It is worth noting too that patients may be neglected at home.

Treatment of the schizophrenic patient is often difficult and unrewarding, but chronicity can be avoided if emphasis is placed on strengthening the patient's ties with reality, i.e. with the community at large, facilitating his or her return to that community as soon as is reasonably possible and avoiding conditions of social neglect. There is much evidence to suggest that many of the features previously held to be typical of chronic schizophrenia are in fact features of social neglect.

Prognosis

Making an accurate prognosis of schizophrenia is difficult but there are a few useful pointers. The following features may be regarded as good prognostic signs:

1   Acute onset.
2   The presence of psychological or physical precipitants, e.g. childbirth, operations.
3   Normal pre-morbid personality.
4   Stable social background, e.g. close social ties.
5   The presence of affective features.
6   Average or above-average intelligence.

The following are poor prognostic features.

1   Insidious onset.
2   Persistent thought disorder.
3   Asthenic bodily habitus.
4   Presence of flattening of affect.
5   Subnormal intelligence.

References

Bleuler, E. (1950) *The Schizophrenias*. International Universities Press, New York.
Färgemann, P. M. (1963) *Psychogenic Psychoses*. Butterworths, London.
Feighner, J. P., Robins, E., Guze, S. B., Woodruffe, R. E., Winokur, G. & Munro, R. (1972) Diagnostic criteria for use in psychiatric research. *Archives of General Psychiatry*, **26**, 57.
Kräpelin, E. (1913) *Psychiatrie*. Barth, Leipzig.

Further reading

Brockington, I. F., Kendell, R. E. & Leff, J. P. (1978) Definitions of schizophrenia: concordance & predictions of outcome. *Psychological Medicine*, **8**, 387–98.
Fish, F. J. (1976) *Schizophrenia*. John Wright, Bristol.
Goffman, E. (1968) *Asylums*. Pelican, London.
Leff, J. & Vaughn, C. E. (1981) Role of expressed emotion on relapse of schizophrenia. *British Journal of Psychiatry*, **139**, 102–4.
Leonhard, K. (1979) *The Classification of Endogenous Psychoses*. Irvington, New York.
Mellor, C. S. (1970) First rank symptoms of schizophrenia. *British Journal of Psychiatry*, **117**, 15–23.
Praag, H. M. van (1975) *On the Origin of Schizophrenic Psychoses*. De Erven Bohn, Amsterdam.
Schneider, K. (1974) Primary and secondary symptoms in schizophrenia. In Hirsch, S. R. & Shepherd, M. (Eds) *Themes and Variations in European Psychiatry*. John Wright, Bristol.

Chapter 4
Organic Syndromes: Dementia, Delirium and Allied States

Introduction

In 1910 Karl Bonhöffer observed that the signs of intracranial disease are independent of the nature of the pathology and depend only on the *site*, the *extent* and *tempo* (rate of onset or spread) of the lesion.

Disturbances of cerebral function consequent on gross physical or subtle neurochemical damage lead to recognizable disorders which are called 'organic syndromes'. In organic syndromes the predominant impairment is of *cognitive function*. Affective symptoms, anxiety, etc. are purely secondary.

1 *Delirium and allied conditions* are characterized by:
   (a) overactivity
   (b) clouded consciousness } acute delirium;
   (c) hallucinosis
   and
   (d) perplexity
   (e) clouded consciousness } subacute delirium ('confusional state').
   (f) incoherent thought

2 *Dementia*
   (a) Primary, where the cause is unknown and not secondary to some other metabolic or structural disturbance. Good examples of primary dementias are Huntington's chorea and Alzheimer's dementia.
   (b) Secondary, where the cause of dementia is known, e.g. atherosclerosis, producing mutli-infarct dementia, tumour or head injury.

Delirium and subacute delirium

Clinical manifestations

The most striking finding in states of delirium is the *impairment of consciousness*. In acute delirium this is severe—in its mildest form it is found in the feelings of 'muzziness in the head' that people experience in ailments such as influenza.

With impaired consciousness the individual's *awareness* of him or herself and of his or her surroundings is impaired. Also the level of wakefulness may be affected. The delirious child is often alarmingly bright-eyed and chatty, but wakefulness, on the other hand, may be reduced, producing a drowsy appearance. With impaired awareness and recognition of the surroundings is found *poor attention and concentration* so that a patient, when asked, cannot perform simple tasks such as washing or tying his pyjama cord without getting lost halfway through. He *cannot register* the information coming in from his environment so naturally fails in simple memory tests.

Disorientation for time and place is invariably present and severe.

Perception is altered, either subtly or grossly. Subtle perceptual alteration is usually first noticed by the patient saying that everything seems clearer and sharper. Later in delirium, *gross perceptual errors* occurs (illusions). When this happens, the patient mistakes patterns on the wallpaper for insects and animals, shadows become menacing people and bedside consultations are heard as sinister plots. Finally the patient experiences *hallucinosis*. Visual hallucinations are common in delirium. They can take many forms. Perhaps the most common are small objects moving quickly across the visual field, e.g. in alcoholic delirium tremens patients often see small animals crawling all over the room. Hallucinations of this sort are described vividly by the patient and frequently appear clearly in his field of vision. Even their bizarre appearance is greeted without surprise, for instance a patient recovering from chronic barbiturate intoxication saw a 6-inch tall manikin running around the room and hiding under floorboards. She identified it as her husband but could not understand why no one would let her prise up the floorboards to let him out. When prevented she became homicidally violent.

Motor disturbance in delirium varies from overactivity in acute delirium to mild irritability seen in subacute delirium. The severe overactivity can be prolonged and exhausting and represents a considerable physical hazard to the patient. The patient is restless, particularly at night, will not stay in bed, and is found wandering about the ward peering out of windows, searching and muttering to him or herself. He or she insists on leaving the ward, must go to work, makes a collection of belongings and arranges and rearranges them, but such is his or her incoherent thinking that it all gets in a muddle and he or she starts all over again.

Emotional symptoms are common. States of panic and terror are usually abrupt in onset, the patient acting under the influence of a misperception of his or her environment. *Milder emotional symptoms* are often missed; this is unfortunate because if recognized they are useful signposts. The mildly delirious patient feels *vaguely apprehensive and uncomfortable* and cannot say why. This may be noticed by the nurses who are surprised to find Mr X unusually uncooperative, having refused his supper.

Delusional ideas in delirium are loose and unformulated and come from the chaotic perceptions that the patient experiences. They never have the clarity and conviction of true schizophrenic delusions.

Physical examination of the delirious patient may reveal common causes such as: (i) alcohol withdrawal; and (ii) pneumonia.

The delirious state itself induces secondary physical changes as the patient refuses food and fluids and so may show signs of: (i) dehydration; (ii) vitamin depletion; and (iii) further psychological disturbance, so that a vicious circle is set up.

Diagnosis

The diagnosis of delirium is not difficult to make providing the examiner concentrates on establishing the state of consciousness and orientation for time and place. Impairment of consciousness and orientation do not occur in schizophrenia nor in mania.

Acute delirium is usually transient, subacute delirious states may last for weeks.

Dementia

Clinical manifestations

In dementia there is *progressive and irreversible intellectual deterioration* consequent to brain damage. The damaged brain cannot absorb and store new information and this is manifest by *impairment of recent memory* which is usually the most striking finding. Patients may complain of this memory defect or it may be noticed by others and not mentioned by the patient. Often patients attempt to overcome this memory defect by keeping a notebook reminding them to do things; this is usually successful for a while but sooner or later the problem overwhelms them and they become anxious and bewildered, fogged by a day's routine which they cannot recall. *Behaviour* shows a deterioration: *interest, activity* and *energy* decline; the professional man copes less easily with his work; the housewife cannot keep up with her chores; the gas is turned on but not lit. Unusual behaviour, e.g. masturbation, self-exposure, shoplifting, can appear as a release phenomenon and with its attendant legal consequences bring about the recognition of the underlying process. The *appearance* deteriorates, clothes become unkempt and stained with food. The decline is overall, leading ultimately to helpless incontinence. *Concentration* is impaired. This can be elicited easily by simple tests such as the serial subtraction of 7 from 100. The patient is often aware of his poor ability and becomes very upset, angry, tearful and agitated when he is confronted with a task which proves too much for him. This is called the *catastrophic reaction*.

The fundamental impairment of brain function in organic brain disease is well demonstrated when this occurs. Organic brain disease produces rigidity of thinking, impairment of grasp and consequent difficulty in problem solving. Psychological tests of brain damage are designed to search for this sort of dysfunction and also to demonstrate difficulty in shifting from abstract to concrete and vice versa.

Emotional changes

There are no specific emotional disturbances. They tend to reflect in an exaggerated form the individual's previous patterns of emotional display. Lability of mood is common as control weakens and in advanced dementia one finds states of 'emotional incontinence'. Depression is common and usually ascribed to the patient's awareness of his plight. *Hysterical symptoms* may appear early in a dementing process. It is suggested that they are caused by the lower order of central nervous control and integration brought about by brain damage.

Diagnosis

The diagnosis of dementia is not difficult when the clinical picture is typical. However, there are difficulties, particularly when confronted with middle-aged patients in whom dementia may be suspected purely on the grounds of a history, say, of declining interest and energy, or many months with some associated mood change. In such a case chronic depression may account for the whole illness, but this may not be so, and one may be left with a patient whom one has to keep under observation.

Aetiology of dementia and delirium

Having found signs of an organic mental state, one is next concerned with finding the underlying cause. The commonest factors causing organic mental syndromes include:

1 Cerebral hypoxia:
   (a) dementia following multiple infarcts gradually depriving the brain of oxygen;
   (b) dementia following prolonged coma, e.g. after carbon monoxide poisoning;
   (c) delirium following cerebral haemorrhage;
   (d) delirium associated with severe pernicious anaemia.
2 Dehydration and electrolyte imbalance:
   (a) delirium due to post-operative fluid loss;
   (b) delirium in uraemia.
3 Vitamin deficiency:
   (a) Wernicke's encephalopathy;
   (b) alcoholic delirium tremens.
4 Chronic intoxications:
   (a) barbiturates;
   (b) alcohol: alcoholic dementia.
5 Gross cerebral damage:
   (a) tumour;
   (b) chronic inflammation: general paralysis;
   (c) head injury causing post-traumatic delirium and dementia.

Investigation of organic syndromes

Physical examination may reveal the cause of delirium or dementia, and may reveal localizing cerebral signs. Commonly, however, physical examination is negative, particularly in cases of dementia, so one employs laboratory and other investigations to clarify the picture. They include:

1 Venereal Disease Research Laboratory (VDRL) investigations, rapid plasma reagin test (RPR), fluorescent treponemal antibody test (FTA);
2 skull X-ray;
3 electroencephalogram (EEG);
4 CSF examination;

5   computerized tomography (CT) brain scan; and
6   cerebral angiography.

Treatment of organic syndromes

General measures

Delirium

The patient should be nursed in quiet surroundings with minimal interference. Calm doctors and nurses reassure the frightened delirious patient and help to maintain contact with reality, however tenuous.

The evening and night are times of heightened overactivity so the patient needs adequate sedation. It is wise to avoid using barbiturates and paraldehyde which may worsen confusion and produce discomfort. Phenothiazine tranquillizers can be given with safety. Diet and fluid should be kept up to the required level and symptomatic treatment with high doses of vitamins is usually given. This should take the form of intravenous parentrovite, 10 ml given 4-hourly for 24 hours, then reduced to 10 ml twice daily intravenously for 24 hours and then 4 ml intramuscularly daily for 5 days.

Dementia

The first thing is to find out the extent of the patient's disability so that one can provide an environment which is stimulating enough to prevent too rapid deterioration but not too demanding. Vitamin B, taken orally, is usually given, though the value of this is doubtful.

Occupational therapy and social therapy have a limited though supportive part to play by providing stimulation and preventing social deterioration.

Special measures

In the treatment of delirium and dementia special measures depend on the nature of the underlying disorder if any—for example, adequate antisyphilitic treatment.

Some special examples of organic syndromes

Conditions caused by vitamin deficiency

1   *Korsakov syndrome*. This may be caused by thiamine deficiency, as in alcoholism, or it can be caused by tumour, cerebral trauma and general metabolic disturbance. The clinical picture includes polyneuritis with the following psychiatric symptoms:

(a)   gross impairment of recent memory;
(b)   confabulation; and
(c)   disorientation.

This type of organic picture is usually called the dysmnesic syndrome.

Typically the patient claims recognition of the doctor and describes the previous meeting in detail, when in fact they have never seen each other before, or will recount in detail the fancied happenings of the previous day—

confabulation. Recent memory is so poor that though the patient may just have been told the examiner's name, he or she is unable to recollect it a minute later. The onset usually follows delirium tremens. The prognosis for complete recovery is bad.

2 *Wernicke's encephalopathy.* This is caused by thiamine deficiency and is found in severe alcoholism or any state of severe malnutrition. Onset of delirium is often sudden and associated with abnormal pupils, ophthalmoplegia and nystagmus.

3 *Pellagra.* Pellagra is caused by a mixed deficiency of tryptophan and niacin. Psychiatric abnormalities may be diverse, ranging from a neurotic to a psychotic picture, but inevitably a frank organic syndrome emerges. This is usually delirium and, untreated, proceeds to dementia, coma and death.

Cardiovascular disease

1 *Cardiac failure.* Patients in cardiac failure are often subject to bouts of mild confusion or subacute delirium at night. This is caused by relative cerebral hypoxia and responds to further treatment of the cardiac condition.

2 *Multi-infarct dementia.* In cerebral arteriosclerosis the onset is earlier than in senile dementia. A typical presentation is episodic with fits and strokes, usually with complete recovery and then a picture of failing memory, concentration and personality change. Stepwise deterioration is the rule.

3 *Thrombosis of the internal carotid artery.* Occlusion of the internal carotid arteries can give rise to dementia usually complicated by focal cerebral signs. A typical history would include transient losses of power in one or other limbs occurring over a period of months followed by gradual alteration in memory.

Cerebral syphilis (general paralysis of the insane)

Now that syphilis is properly treated in its early stages, the full-blown picture of general paralysis of the insane (GPI) is rarely seen. The first signs of GPI are usually those of sudden personality change, with radical alteration of the patient's previous ethical and moral standards. This is followed by grandiose and extravagant behaviour. After this the picture settles into one of dementia with failing memory and general deterioration. The affective state is usually one of flat euphoria. Spastic paralysis, pupillary abnormalities and physical deterioration are late manifestations.

Syndromes following head injury

Dementia can follow severe head injury, as can fits, which are a common sequel of head injury of whatever severity.

Traumatic dementia usually follows extensive destruction of brain tissue. States of delirium with complete recovery can also follow severe head injury.

The term *post-contusional syndrome* is usually applied to a constellation of mild chronic symptoms including headache, dizziness and general feelings of weakness and inability to concentrate. This syndrome is regarded as being constitutionally determined and released by injury. Post-contusional syndromes can present difficult problems in management. In general it is advisable for patients to return to normal life and work as soon as reasonably possible since it has been found that prolonged unnecessarily convalescence delays rehabilitation and fixes neurotic symptoms. The morale of patients is always improved by confident management, maximum reassurance and vigorous rehabilitation.

Other dementias

Alzheimer's disease (senile dementia)

The original description of Alzheimer's disease was of a pre-senile dementia but it has for some time been realized that the symptoms and pathology found in Alzheimer's pre-senile dementia and 'senile dementia' are similar, so that now it is customary to refer to this type of dementia—the most common of all—as Alzheimer's disease and when it occurs in the older age groups as senile dementia (Alzheimer type).

Commonly the first manifestations of Alzheimer's disease are exaggeration of the basic changes of ageing, namely increased rigidity of thinking, greater egocentricity and lessened emotional control. These exaggerations may precede the appearance of frank evidence of dementia. Sometimes not for years, but inevitably, memory impairment, poor concentration and impaired performance show themselves, while the individual's social behaviour becomes less tolerable. Important findings to look for include apraxia, aphasia, and agraphia which are inevitable accompaniments of the disorder. Neglect of the self, appearance and so on become more marked, all the mental powers enter a decline and individuals with the disease end up as an empty shell of their former selves, incontinent, helpless, incapable of grasping what is going on around them.

In Alzheimer's disease motor and parietal symptoms are prominent with severe fall-out in the hippocampal region. There is increase in muscle tone, unsteadiness of gait and spatial disorientation. The process is more gradual than atheromatous dementia. The possibility of pseudodementia should never be overlooked. In this the most common cause in the elderly is an unrecognized depressive state which usually responds very well to antidepressant treatment.

Creutzfeldt's disease

This is an acute, viral panencephalitis known variously as Kuru (in Papua), scrapie (in sheep), and spongiform encephalopathy (in cattle). It is characterized by onset in middle life with ataxia, myoclonus and rapidly progressing dementia leading to stupor and death within a few months.

Pick's disease

In this condition an hereditary cerebral atrophy is mainly confined to the frontal and temporal poles, so that commonly its presentation is as a frontal lobe syndrome with impaired moral standards. It is a rare dementia sometimes manifesting itself as early as the fifth decade of life. Amnesia and progressive dementia are particularly prominent and motor and parietal symptoms are comparatively less common. With the passage of time, however, the clinical picture becomes indistinguishable from Alzheimer's disease.

Huntington's chorea

This is a genetically determined form of dementia. The inheritance is caused by dominant genes. The manifestations of Huntington's chorea are choreiform movements and altered mental states leading inevitably to dementia. A wide range of psychiatric symptomatology may be seen before dementia becomes evident, although the most commonly found psychoses are paranoid in type. Suicide, alcoholism and personality disorders are common in Huntington families.

Psychiatric aspects of epilepsy

The fact is often overlooked that being epileptic is an extremely frightening and theatening experience. The knowledge that one may suddenly, without warning, have total loss of consciousness is an extremely distressing one for patient and family alike. For this reason the epileptic patient needs, in addition to proper anti-convulsant therapy, sensible support and guidance so that he or she may be enabled to live as normal a life as possible without 'wrapping the patient in cotton wool', which can easily happen with epileptic children. The important special psychiatric aspects of epilepsy concern temporal lobe epilepsy and epileptic psychoses. In temporal lobe epilepsy (TLE) episodic mood disturbances or outbursts or rage may often be associated with the epileptic discharge and accompanied by appropriate EEG changes. Sometimes TLE may pass unrecognized because the emotional disturbance, whether it is rage, ecstasy or perceptual disturbance, somehow overshadows the seizure-related aspect of the disorder. It should always be considered when presented with a patient who has an episodic type of behaviour disturbance or mood change.

The association of epilepsy with psychosis is an interesting one. For some time it was thought that there was a negative correlation between schizophrenia and epilepsy. In fact, this is not true. There is a definite association between epilepsy and schizophreniform psychoses and the current view is that these are symptomatic psychoses, i.e. psychoses which originate in the epileptic process and are not independent of it. There is a high correlation between temporal lobe epilepsy and the development of epileptic psychoses.

In the past, personality changes were described in long-standing, poorly-controlled epileptic patients. The changes noted included tendencies towards rigidity, seclusiveness and rather difficult behaviour. These changes are uncommon and were probably related to prolonged stay in institutions plus the effects of taking excessive medication. Perhaps the only association between epilepsy and personality change is an apparent association, at least, between temporal lobe epilepsy and personality disorder.

Syndromes associated with cerebral tumour

The common modes of presentation of cerebral tumour are:
1   epilepsy;
2   signs of raised intracranial pressure, e.g. headache, papilloedema, nausea, vertigo; and

3 manifestations of local or generalized brain damage, e.g. dysphasia, apraxia, dementia, paresis.

However, it is not uncommon for tumours to present with apparently 'pure' psychiatric symptoms. Even more misleading can be the occurrence of tumour in a patient with long-standing neurotic complaints. In either instance if the doctor is not alert the diagnosis will be missed until signs of gross damage appear.

Probably about 50% of patients with cerebral tumour present in this way, i.e. with psychiatric symptomatology. This places a critical diagnostic burden on anyone evaluating such symptoms, particularly in children and in patients of middle age who are most at risk from tumour development.

The following manifestations should always be enquired about most carefully and evaluated:

1 subtle, insidious personality change
2 deterioration in appearance
3 altered ethical and moral standards
4 recent affective flattening, insouciance and apathy ⎬ point to frontal lobe tumours;

5 unusual flippancy
6 poor concentration
7 memory impairment
8 hallucinations ⎬ point to temporal lobe tumours;

9 bouts of sleepiness ⎬ point to third ventricle tumours.

Narcolepsy is a rare cause of bouts of sleepiness with a characteristic EEG. It responds to amphetamines.

Reference
Bonhöffer, K. (1910) *Die symptomatischen Psychosen in Gefolge von akuten Infectionen und innere Erkrankungen.* Deuticke, Leipzig.

Further reading
Bonhöffer, K. (1974) Exogenous psychoses. In Hirsch, S. R. & Shepherd, M. (Eds) *Themes and Variations in European Psychiatry.* John Wright, Bristol.

Flohr-Henry, P. (1976) Epilepsy and psychopathology. *Recent Advances in Clinical Psychiatry,* **2,** 262–95.

Keschner, M., Bender, M. B. & Strauss, I. (1938) Mental symptoms associated with brain tumor. *Journal of the American Medical Association,* **110,** 714–18.

Lishman, W. A. (1987) *Organic Psychiatry.* Blackwell Scientific Publications, Oxford.

Luria, A. R. (1980) *Higher Cortical Functions in Man.* Basic Books, New York.

Luria, A. R. (1989) *The Working Brain.* Penguin, London.

Slater, E., Beard, A. W. & Clithero, E. (1963) The schizophrenic psychoses of epilepsy. *British Journal of Psychiatry,* **109,** 95.

Symonds, C. (1962) Concussion and its sequelae. Lancet, i, 1.

Wolff, H. G. & Curran, D. (1935) The nature of delirium and allied states; dysergastic reaction. *Archives of Neurology and Psychiatry (Chicago),* **33,** 1175–215.

Chapter 5
Neurosis and Personality Disorders

Introduction

The disease concept in psychiatry is strongest as far as the organic psychoses are concerned. In these disorders, structural brain pathology produces recognizable psychiatric syndromes. The concept is less strong in the case of the functional psychoses, i.e. *schizophrenia* and *manic depressive psychosis*, though evidence of *biochemical disturbance* is impressive. In the case of the neuroses and personality disorders, this concept is at its weakest since these conditions are quantitative differences from the normal, as opposed to specific disorders such as the organic and functional psychoses.

Neurotic depression and anxiety can be triggered off by many causes and are often found in people with vulnerable or abnormal personalities. This means that neurosis and personality disorder are interwoven. Many find it difficult to accept personality disorder as an *illness* because personality disorders do not represent a change in an individual any more than does being ugly or beautiful—that is how the person is!

Concept of personality

In order to deal with variation in the character of people, psychiatrists face a daunting problem in finding a model that is finite yet does justice to the unique nature of the infinity of characters that compose the human world. To treat each case as wholly unique, with no learning nor generalization from previous patients acceptable, means one might just as well consult anyone. Yet to pigeon-hole people arbitrarily into one of a few groups is surely to lose sight of much of what makes a person what he or she is.

To capture this infinite variety in a way one can handle, consider the measurement of any psychological dimension, e.g. intelligence (Fig. 1). The average of the *healthy* population is defined as 100 points. One standard deviation (mean of difference of each person's score from the average) is about 15 points. Two-thirds of the population fall within 1 standard deviation (S.D.) from 100. All but 3% of the population fall within 2 S.D., i.e. IQ between 70 and 130 points. People outside this range are deviant, maybe abnormal. Analogously any psychological variable may be measured by arbitrary construction of an 'instrument' (usually a questionaire). It is then tested for *reliability* and *validity*. For example, an IQ test is not *reliable* if the results obtained by different observers from the same patient are different. A test may not measure what it purports to measure: for example, an IQ test may not test intelligence but merely the ability to fill in forms. In that case, the test is not *valid*.

Shyness is a trait often correlated with sensitive personality. It illustrates the continuity from the average to very deviant experience that is part of the

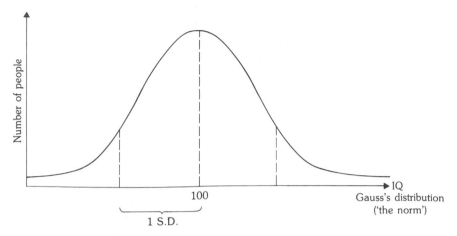

Fig. 1 Intelligence range of the average population.

normal range of any personality characteristic. School assemblies may be remembered for the occasional child fainting and the subsequent tiresome discussions as to whether it was too hot or too cold. Research found, however, that the children usually fainted (regardless of temperature) during 'head-master's announcements'. These were sometimes mildly unpleasant affairs where accusatory remarks were uttered, such as 'Someone has stolen some books from the library'. Fleeting feelings of guilt occur when the child feels the headmaster is referring to him or her; indeed such feelings are normally (Gaussianly) distributed in the population. The sensitive child, feeling the headmaster's gaze and the eyes of the school on the back of his or her neck, flushes and, rarely, faints. Such people show an exceptional tendency to construe general statements as personally directed. When grown up, these individuals are the sort who may think that people laughing at a table in a pub when they enter are laughing at them. Such a person would be described as a sensitive personality disorder if, for example, he or she presented with alcoholism due to drinking to dissolve these unpleasant feelings.

Consider now a three-dimensional version of Gauss's curve, a Guassian hillock, which will look rather like a Mexican hat (Fig. 2). From above (i.e. in plan) the Guassian 'hillock of personality' is the figure of a circle. Any vertical section through the centre of the hillock is a diameter of the circle. In elevation, the edge cut between the hillock surface and the vertical section is the shape of Gauss's curve. The cut represents any psychological dimension such as obsessionality, shyness, sensitivity, etc. An infinite number of diameters may be drawn on the circle, each quantifying a characteristic known as a psychological dimension of personality. This *nomothetic*, or statistical approach, comple-ments the *ideographic* approach of literature. We say one 'measures person-ality', the other 'describes character'.

Many psychometric tests are named after their inventors and their acronyms often end in I' for 'inventory'. The Millon Clinical Multiaxial Inventory (MCMI) is a bank of tests of several psychological dimensions used to produce a

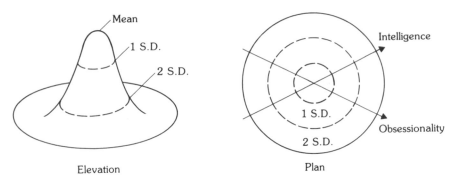

Fig. 2 The Gaussian 'hillock of personality'.

personality profile. It provides a reliable and valid analysis of personality (Fig. 3). Note that the patient whose psychometry on the 'sensitive' dimension is more than 2 standard deviations away from the mean is either a paranoic or merely very sensitive, but 'normal' (i.e. part of the distribution) just as a man who is 6′ 7″ tall has either a pituitary disorder or is very tall, but 'normal'.

In the consideration of how personality is scientifically modelled, the word 'abnormal' was used in its strict statistical sense, i.e. *qualitatively* distinct from anything in the normal (i.e. Gaussian) distribution. However, 'abnormal' is used throughout the literature on personality disorder in its vernacular meaning to indicate deviation from the average. This unfortunate loss of clarity cannot be avoided, but it may help to remember that 'abnormal personality' is the sort found, for example, in schizophrenic disintegration. In the next section, 'abnormal' is used in the loose sense of 'deviant'.

Abnormal personality and psychopathy

Many people behave abnormally from their earliest years. This abnormality can show itself in antisocial acts, addiction, social inadequacy, undue vulnerability or

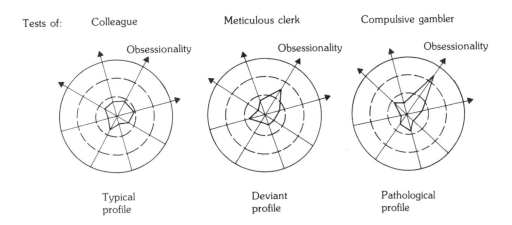

Fig. 3 Personality profiles using MCMI tests.

in eccentricity of one sort or another. It is part of their constitution rather than an acquired illness, and for this reason is ascribed to their having abnormal personalities. *Personality* is the sum of many different varying characteristics, intellectual, affective and physical, to name only a few, which gives to each person both an individuality and a resemblance to his or her fellows. These characteristics are present to some degree in everyone, so that to speak of *normal* and *abnormal* personality is not to postulate endpoints separating the two categories, but rather to define an individual's personality as lying somewhere along a curve of normal distribution. In this way, the abnormals are those who deviate markedly from the average and the normals are the bulk of the population. This method of considering personality has the great advantage of being experimentally valuable. Investigators can then go further and attempt to establish the psychological correlates of given personality characteristics. Much valuable work of this sort has already been carried out. The psychiatric approach to the study of *abnormal personalities* has in the main been a clinical one and has not been made easy to follow by the use of the term *psychopath*.

In general, psychiatrists have tended to call psychopaths those patients with abnormal personalities, but this is not universally so. The two concepts of psychopathy and personality disorder were most succinctly united by Schneider (1958) who defined psychopaths as *those abnormal personalities who suffer from their abnormality or cause society to suffer*. This definition is the one used in this book. It has one very important advantage, namely that it recognizes that someone can have an abnormal ('abaverage' or 'deviant', to be statistically correct) personality without being regarded in some way as ill or antisocial, i.e. distinguishes between 'pathological' and 'non-pathological' abnormal personalities. This is important because the term psychopath has come to be regarded, in Anglo-American circles anyway, almost as a term of abuse. Unfortunately the picture (in England and Wales) has been made more complicated by the Mental Health Act of 1959, in which the definition of psychopathic disorder stresses irresponsible or antisocial conduct.

Psychiatrists have classified psychopaths in two main ways; first by naming groups whose personality disorder resembles a clinical syndrome, e.g. schizoid psychopath, hysterical psychopath and secondly, by naming groups descriptively, e.g. inadequate psychopath, aggressive psychopath. These classifications are convenient shorthands for reducing the infinite variety somewhat arbitrarily to large groups (Fig. 4). Though convenient, such categories as 'inadequate' are no substitute for a perceptive thumb-nail sketch of character. Such vignettes are important for illustrating the target of treatment and the International Classification of Diseases (ICD) categories are such vignettes of the commonest presentations.

Variations of abnormal personalities

Non-pathological ('deviant')

Many people of undoubted genius fall into this category. Some authorities would call them psychopaths but there seems no justification for this.

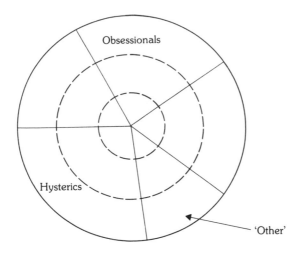

The 'infinite variety of diameters' (particularly personality characteristics) are shrunk to a few 'cake-wedges' (clinically common categories)

Fig. 4 Classification of psychopaths.

Pathological (psychopaths)

The abnormalities which cause symptoms include:

1 hypochondria

2 instability

3 lability of mood

4 abuse of drugs

may lead to admission to hospital.

The abnormalities which offend society include:

1 suicidal gestures

2 antisocial behaviour—recidivism

3 lack of foresight leading to gratification of any need

4 explosive behaviour

5 sexual perversions

6 social inadequacy

7 inability to maintain stable interpersonal relationships

may lead to hospital, or more commonly, to prison.

The striking feature of so many psychopaths is their *remarkable degree of immaturity* of personality development. They react to the whim of the moment in much the same way as does a small child who has tantrums if his or her wishes are not gratified immediately. The same sort of thing leads them into crimes which can have disastrous consequences.

Treatment

Just as one cannot alter one's height and the leopard cannot change his spots, no treatment can transform someone's personality. But if the leopard cannot change his spots, at least he can know he has them and make any necessary allowances for them. A very tall man presenting with headaches because he keeps bumping his head on the door frame has to learn to stoop, to enlarge the door frames or move to a house with tall doors. First, however, he has to under-stand and accept the origin of his headaches. Treatment of the psychopath is similar. He or she may be given insight, and this is most efficiently done by group psychotherapy where patients can knock the spots off each other. The display of psychopathic behaviour by others is a way such patients can objectively observe what the doctor is trying to treat. The approach to the patient acknowledges the importance of social forces and of the therapeutic community as a whole in influencing behaviour. Contrary to popular belief, psychopaths can do well with such treatment.

The neuroses

In the classification of neuroses (300) and personality disorders (301) in the international classification of disease, it quickly becomes apparent that the same labels are used for both, e.g. 'obsessional neurosis' (300.3), 'obsessional personality disorder' (301.4). This is because a person deviant along one particular dimension will tend to decompensate under stress by becoming more deviant in that dimension. This 'psychic strain' is called a *neurosis*, the meticulous, fastidious character becomes pedantic and obsessional. If psycholo-gists had developed tools sufficiently sensitive (and reliable and valid!) we might find the results of Fig. 5 on investigation.

The deterioration in the obsessional score (i.e. the psychic strain under the stress of unemployment) to more than 2 S.D. and its relief on gaining work show that, phenomenologically, neurosis can be likened to temporary patho-logical personality. A general concept of neurosis identifies it as a psychological disorder characterized by:

1   the absence of symptoms such as hallucinations, delusions, thought disorder or intellectual impairment;
2   the presence of anxiety;

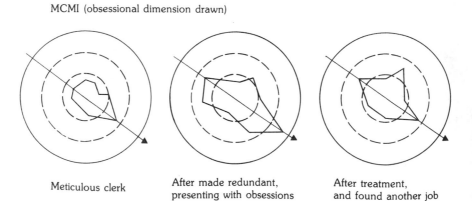

MCMI (obsessional dimension drawn)

Meticulous clerk   After made redundant, presenting with obsessions   After treatment, and found another job

Fig. 5 Patterns of deviance in the classification of neurosis.

3 mild chronic symptoms;
4 *preservation of insight*; and
5 no change in personality.
as opposed to the psychoses' severe disorders characterized by:
1 manifestations such as hallucinations, delusions, thought disorder and intellectual impairment;
2 severe mood disturbance;
3 *poor insight*;
4 relative absence of anxiety; and
5 personality change.

The neuroses are common disorders and account for 20–25% of patients attending general practitioners. The neuroses covered here include the following:
1 anxiety;
2 hysteria;
3 obsessional disorder; and
4 hypochondriasis.

Anxiety

Anxiety is a universal phenomenon in which the subject experiences a feeling *akin to fear or apprehension* usually accompanied by autonomic disturbances (sympathetic overactivity), of which the following are typical:
1 tachycardia and raised blood pressure;
2 palpitations;
3 dryness of mouth;
4 diarrhoea, epigastric discomfort, nausea;
5 dilated pupils;
6 sweating;
7 frequency of micturition; and
8 headaches.

Despite its universality, not all anxiety is pathological. It is useful to distinguish between *healthy* and *morbid* anxiety.

Healthy anxiety is experienced by most people, unaccustomed *stress*—examinations, interviews, etc.—being typical examples. It is a normal response to an unusual situation, an *adaptive response* on the part of the organism which prepares the subject for a task or ordeal requiring further effort and making unusual demands on him or her.

Morbid anxiety, however, is different; it is a *maladaptive response* and serves no useful purpose, once it is established—quite the opposite in fact! Too often it pervades the mental life of the individual and becomes a rein, not a spur. The morbidly anxious patient is soon aware of the *paradoxical nature* of his or her affliction. Anxiety is experienced both in the presence of, or the absence of what can be seen to be obvious stimuli. The patient knows that these fears are irrational and groundless but nevertheless helplessly magnifies, scrutinizes and mulls over the content of his or her anxiety.

Aetiology

Age

Anxiety is common in adolescence and old age. *Adolescence* can be and often is a time of stress and turmoil. Young people are subject to all sorts of pressures at this time of their lives. Normal adolescent development is a period during which strong emotions are easily aroused—emotions which subjects find hard to channel. They are at an 'in between' stage of life where they are accorded neither adult nor childish status. The adolescent is often oversensitive and prickly, particularly about his or her appearance, which is more often than not gauche and pimply. It is hardly surprising then that emergent sexuality is tantalized by advertisements extolling the virtues of flawless skin or correct bust size. The adolescent is full of self-doubt. Will he or she get a job? The right sort of job? Will he or she get into university? Will he or she be socially, sexually and in every other way competent when put to the test? All these sorts of questions are in the adolescent's mind and it seems that everyone offers conflicting advice. In this setting he or she may develop *anxiety symptoms*, usually of an acute sort.

Often the anxiety symptoms of the adolescent may find their most extreme expression in a near psychotic breakdown—sometimes mistakenly diagnosed as schizophrenia—which has been called the *adolescent crisis of identity*. This syndrome is really what the name suggests, a state in which youngsters become so uncertain of themselves and their role that they break down into an overwhelming state of anxious uncertainty where contact with reality may apparently be lost. A good fictional description of this is to be found in the novel *Catcher in the Rye* by J. D. Salinger.

The adolescent crisis of identity usually responds well to straightforward and sympathetic management. It is important that such patients are not mistakenly *labelled* as schizophrenic; on the other hand it has to be remembered that schizophrenia is a state which can and does begin in adolescence. But in schizophrenia the evidence for a more profound process should be sought for: personality change, thought disorder, etc. (see 'Schizophrenia', p. 24).

Sources of anxiety in adolescence then are common; they may be personal, social or cultural. The symptom itself needs investigation and treatment since adolescence is a time of change and maturation. Sensible handling in adolescence may help the individual avoid chronicity of symptoms and the carrying over of unresolved adolescent problems into adult life.

Elderly people readily become anxious when the orderly routine of their life is threatened. Loneliness and the fear of death are also important causes of anxiety in old age. Often the anxieties of the elderly may be too readily dismissed as if they were of little significance because the patient is *old*, as if old age were necessarily a sort of *laissez-passer* to wretchedness, which it need not be though too often is.

Constitution—the anxious personality

Some people are, by nature, more anxious than others. From early years and throughout their lives they are insecure, timid and emotionally unstable. They are tense, their fears are easily aroused and they are over fussy about their health—tending readily towards hypochondriasis. Their *work records are poor*, and they show a *low level of drive, energy, ambition* and *persistence*. This combination of traits is regarded as evidence of *constitutional neuroticism* and the evidence for its existence has been convincingly demonstrated (Slater, 1943; Rees & Eysenck, 1945). Neuroticism correlates highly with physique, vaso-motor instability and a background of poor general health.

Anxiety neurosis (neurotic decompensation)

Anxiety is probably the commonest form of psychic strain in response to psychic stresses. To an extent this is a normal but self-limiting response, e.g. before exams, getting married, fighting. If it persists there is usually a persisting stress factor that must be removed if the anxiety is to resolve.

Learning

There is much experimental evidence to suggest that anxiety is sometimes a learned phenomenon, i.e. it has been developed by a process of simple conditioning, and is subject to the same laws (generalization, inhibition, extinction, etc.) This has been exploited therapeutically by using processes of *deconditioning* to extinguish *phobias* (see p. 60).

Clinical manifestations

In addition to experiencing the specific manifestations described at the beginning of this section, anxious patients often complain of feelings of *tension*, or of difficulty in *concentrating*. Tension manifests itself not only by a 'feeling of being strung up' but also by heaviness or pains in the limbs.

Associated *mood change of depressive type* is very commonly associated with anxiety—in fact, a state of anxiety in pure culture is extremely rare—sooner or later depression appears.

Other bodily accompaniments of anxiety include decreased libido and impotence. Sleep is poor—typically patients find it hard to get off to sleep and may experience broken sleep throughout the night, when they will tend to lie awake worrying about their fears.

Anxiety states may present to the doctor in a wide range of symptoms involving almost every system of the body: the cardiologist may be consulted about palpitations; the chest physician about difficulty in breathing; the gastroenterologist about dyspepsia and the neurologist about weakness and headaches. The bodily manifestations of anxiety are likely to be those of which the patient complains, since they are what make him or her feel unwell. While careful investigation is a part of all medical care, it has to be realized in the treat-ment of the patient suffering from anxiety that investigation carried to excess may reinforce the disorder. The doctor has to strike a balance between over-investigation with inadequate reassurance and under-investigation with overconfident reassurance.

Diagnosis

Simple states of anxiety uncomplicated by depression are uncommon. Most anxious patients have some depressive mood change. Anxiety may be prominent in the onset of a depressive illness. It is also not uncommon to find anxiety in the early stages of schizophrenia. Before deciding that a patient is suffering from simple anxiety one has to exclude:

1   depression; and
2   schizophrenia.

However, episodic attacks which can be confused with anxiety can be caused by:

1   temporal lobe epilepsy;
2   adrenaline secreting tumours; and
3   hypoglycaemia.

It is useful to distinguish whether episodic autonomic symptoms such as panic attacks presenting, for example, as the patient being housebound, dominate the clinical picture, or whether chronic tension is more prominent. The former (panics) is often just faulty learning, with crowds, buses, or whatever being the mental clothes peg upon which the patient has hung the explanation of tachycardia, hyperventilation, etc. The latter (tension) may be a personality trait or a decompensating strain in the face of some social stress.

Treatment

The treatment is psychological. Only where anxiety is so overwhelming that it prevents the patient's cooperation is a brief initial sedation with a benzodiazepine (Diazepam, up to 60 mg per day reducing to zero after 2 weeks) appropriate. Beta blockers are helpful with symptoms such as tremors, but they make psychological treatment more difficult.

Anxious personality

Surprising though it may seem, it is possible to gain some degree of voluntary control over most autonomic functions, even over the alpha rhythm of the electroencephalogram. Learning how to do this provides a constructive channel for the energy of the anxious patient. Traditionally this method has been put to use by oriental ascetic mystics and it finds its modern manifestation in the popularity of yoga, zen and various meditations.

Biofeedback is the distilled technical essential of all these methods. One of the most efficient forms is a click-feedback of the skin resistance. Two sponge electrodes wrapped round two fingers are connected to a galvanometer. As the patient relaxes and sweats less, skin resistance rises, less current can flow through the meter, triggering fewer of the Geigercounter-like 'clicks'. The patient simply has to lower the frequency of the clicks, and quickly notices the effect of relaxing muscles, breathing more slowly but deeply, etc. Modes of thought—hurried, reflective, etc.—also influence the rate of feedback and effectively educate the patient, giving him or her insight into the nature of tension and methods of symptomatically reducing it.

Neurotic anxiety

Where the stress is identifiable (e.g. marital, family, economic), amelioration, even if only ventilation, is helpful and logical. Benzodiazepines, while symptomatically helpful, aggravate the situation by decreasing psychomotor efficiency (by over 40% on testing). They are disinhibiting for the same reason that alcohol is, and so can make the patient more volatile. They are also cumulative and addictive.

The simplest form of psychotherapy is supportive. In this the doctor listens and permits the patient to ventilate his or her feelings and arrive at solutions of problems without guidance or interpretation. The role of the doctor is to provide unbiased sympathy and encouragement. Analytic psychotherapy may be helpful if the anxiety is secondary to past traumas.

For faulty learning, cognitive therapy is the most successful treatment. When anxiety is linked to specific stresses (e.g. cats, heights, open spaces) and triggered off by these, it is called *phobic anxiety*. These phobias may be single or multiple and the triggering stresses may be very vague. In recent years, psychologists studying theories of learning have pointed out that phobias are probably the result of maladaptive learning, i.e. the patient has become conditioned to experience anxiety at the sight or sound of a given object. They have reasoned from this that the phobias could be cured by a deconditioning process which desensitizes the patient to the cause of the attacks. This has the advantage of being based on a rational theoretical basis. By desensitizing, the subject learns to avoid responding to noxious stimuli by being exposed to the stimuli at levels where he or she can manage the response. In this way, he or she becomes inured to the stimuli and the response is lost. 'Flooding' or implosion means the patient is 'thrown in at the deep end' by being brought face to face with the dreaded stimulus until the anxiety fades. To illustrate these principles, the appendix to this chapter is an example of a sheet given to outpatients being treated for phobias.

Hysteria

The word hysteria is used in at least three ways:

1   To describe a variety of abnormal personality, *hysterical personality*.

2   To describe certain disorders, *hysterical neuroses (conversion hysteria)*, in which there is loss of function without organic damage. These disorders are induced by stress and the patient is unconscious of the mechanism.

3   To describe unconscious exaggeration of organic disease, so-called '*hysterical overlay*' or '*hysterical exaggeration*'.

The 'unconscious mechanism' in **2** and **3** is often referred to as the 'secondary gain' the patient obtains from such behaviour.

Hysterical personality (histrionic personality)

The term hysterical personality has been used to describe a personality type characterized by a tendency towards histrionic behaviour. Such individuals show the following traits:

1   Affective immaturity often allied to an appearance of physical immaturity.
2   Egocentricity allied to a remarkable capacity for self deception.
3   Histrionic behaviour. To the hysteric the world is either hell or heaven. Extremes of feeling easily aroused and as easily dissipated are commonplace. This is reflected in their appearance in striking fashion. At one moment such patients can be ashen-faced, weeping wrecks threatening suicide, disrupting the whole atmosphere of the ward; hours later, or less, they are the most vivacious and sought-after partners at the hospital dance.
4   Inability to tolerate or maintain interpersonal relationships of any depth.

Of course, the hysteric possesses these traits to an excessive degree—they are common enough in normal people. Under certain circumstances the hysterical peronality can be an asset, e.g. in the theatre.

Hysterical neurosis (conversion hysteria)

In hysterical disorders there is loss of function without organic damage. This usually arises as a result of stress in a susceptible person but can occur in otherwise normal individuals in face of overwhelming stress (e.g. disasters, wartime).

The lost function protects the patient from further harm. It may be asked whether the illness is simulated. The answer is yes, but the patient is wholly or partly unaware of this.

With increasing scientific knowledge of the population, hysterical deficits have become less gross and more subtle. Hysterical dysmnesia is now much commoner than hysterical paralysis.

Hysterical disorders are diverse. Most commonly they affect higher functions and the central nervous system producing amnaesia, paralysis, sensory loss, etc. Hysteria can also produce pseudo-dementia in which the patient develops an apparent psychotic state. The signs of 'psychosis' conform to the layman's idea of madness, e.g. when asked how many legs a cow has, a patient might answer 'five'. Pains can be hysterical in origin. When this is so, it is a common error to suppose that the patient is therefore not experiencing discomfort but is feigning. As so little is known about the mechanism of pain there seems no justification for this belief. It is wiser to acknowledge that the patient is in pain and try and discover the cause. Pain is pain whether hysterical or not, and the label hysterical should not be allowed to cause patients to be subjected to the sort of hostile treatment that they may provoke by their admittedly often demanding and rather ruthless behaviour.

Aetiology

1   The role of the hysterical personality has been mentioned. There is strong evidence to support the belief that genetic factors are important in this.
2   It is likely too that upbringing can reinforce already dominant hysterical traits. The doting parent who accedes to every whim of an unstable egocentric child is probably doing this unwittingly.
3   *Brain damage, mental subnormality and chronic psychosis* all predispose to hysteria by lowering higher control and integration.

4   Hysterical disorders are danger signals. The undiagnosed depressive and the incipient schizophrene who finds his or her inner life mysteriously disrupted may both develop hysterical symptoms as an unconscious call for help.

5   The manifestations of hysteria conform to: (a) the patient's notion of illness, thus sensory loss is of 'glove' or 'stocking' distribution; and (b) ideas of disease implanted in the patient's mind by others, either by suggestion or example. Doctors can suggest the former and other patients the latter by their own symptoms.

6   The psychodynamic explanation of hysterical disorder is that the failure in function always arises as a result of unconscious conflict or buried psychic trauma. These threaten the individual's integrity to such an extent that he or she responds by switching off a function, thus making it unnecessary to continue in the stressful situation as he or she is now ill and can opt out. This switching off is referred to as dissociation or secondary gain.

Diagnosis

Since hysteria can mimic so many other illnesses the differential diagnosis is limitless. It should be made on positive and not negative grounds; it is not good enough to investigate a patient's complaints and, having found no abnormality, fall back on hysteria as a convenient dumping ground.

One must have adequate reasons for making the diagnosis, so that one can look at the patient's history and life situation and see with certainty that a hysterical disorder is the inevitable outcome of all that has gone before. There is often discernible 'secondary gain'.

Hysteria is a diagnosis that is often made lightly by the inexperienced, purely on the basis of a few negative results.

Treatment

Hysterical personality disorder

Such patients usually make brief, dramatic appearances in hospital following suicidal gestures, marital strife or any acute stress that is too much for their level of tolerance. Mood disturbances may be prominent but rarely sustained.

Tranquillizing drugs may be needed to calm the patient in a period of acute crisis. The object should be to make the period of hospital stay as short as possible to tide the patient over the crisis. After this treatment either consists of: (i) simple supportive therapy, or (ii) group psychotherapy or transactional analysis (p. 108) aimed at helping the patient towards insight and a higher level of emotional maturity.

Hysterical neurosis (conversion hysteria)

General measures

It is important to treat the patient actively, i.e. to do everything possible that will help to convince him or her that total function will return. At the same time one has to *avoid* focusing too much on the *symptom* and reinforcing it in the patient's mind.

This can be done fairly easily as long as doctors and nurses approach the patient as a team and with full knowledge of each other's roles. Difference of opinion and uncertainty feed hysteria. The patient, sensing differing attitudes, questions different people, gets different answers and the symptoms intensify and proliferate.

Abreaction

Freud used this term to describe the reliving of emotionally charged experiences said to have caused hysterical breakdown. It has a place in the treatment of hysteria but is most successful in the acute disorder, i.e. immediately following some traumatic experience.

Abreaction is encouraged in a state of altered consciousness—usually brought about by giving intravenous sodium amytal (250–500 mg). In theory, the patient regains the lost function once he has ventilated the pent-up feeling that surrounds the traumatic scene. *Hypnosis* where *the patient lets him or herself* relax is psychological abreaction. The drawback of hypnosis or drug-induced abreaction is that the patient has taken no personal responsibility so it induces dependence on the therapist (sadly much liked by some therapists). The patient may get better but learns nothing of how to deal with similar problems and may return again for treatment by 'magic wand'.

Psychotherapy

The alternatives are: (i) supportive therapy, or (ii) exploratory psychotherapy with the object of helping the patient to understand the nature of the illness and how it relates to his or her life situation. This often means embarking on fairly prolonged analytic psychotherapy. Transactional analysis is (p. 108) is helpful.

Obsessional disorders

Obsessions and compulsions are similar though not identical psychological manifestations. Their similarity lies in the fact that they are both experienced against an inner feeling of resistance. Obsessions are contents of consciousness, ideas or thoughts which the patient has but tries to push away. Sometimes they develop into acts, utterances or rituals, and become repetitive, in which case they are called compulsions. In practice they are described collectively by the term obsessive compulsive phenomena.

Aetiology

Normal development

Everyone has experienced the 'tune that keeps running through the head', or the rituals practised in childhood, e.g. walking on paving stones avoiding the lines. These are part of normal life and development and resemble obsessive compulsive phenomena. Children often use these rituals in a magical way to defend themselves from fancied harm. It has been suggested that rituals are used in a similar way in obsessional illness.

Personality type

Some people are from their early years overmeticulous and unduly scrupulous. They show excessive concern for order and tidiness in dress and in their surroundings. Their talk is precise, even pedantic, while their outlook is excessively moral and rigid. They tend to be indecisive, vacillatory and hypochondriacal. Their indecisiveness makes them good subordinates but poor leaders. They lack imagination or creative ability, and humour, when present, is of an arid, donnish sort. Such traits constitute the *obsessional personality*. If such people become psychologically ill, they develop obsessional symptoms. When such individuals develop say, a depressive state, their illness tends to be very much coloured by their personality so that they often present with an interminable kind of pedantic hypochondriacal talk which may mask the depressive mood change which becomes more apparent as the interview proceeds.

Relation to brain damage

1 Obsessional symptoms are definitely associated with the personality changes following encephalitis lethargica.
2 Brain-damaged patients often develop obsessional tidiness, 'organic order-liness'. This can be seen as the way in which progressively handicapped individuals attempt to impose order on an environment that is becoming too much for them.

Manifestations

Obsessional symptoms tend to focus on daily activities such as eating, dressing, washing and defaecation—a patient complained that she was unable to eat as she spent hours removing solid particles from food matter. Another patient never finished her housework as she felt obliged to repeat the washing-up time and time again. A patient could not get to work on time as he was delayed by elaborate rituals surrounding his morning defaecation.

Usually the patient seeks medical advice because the symptoms have *got out of hand*. They have usually been present for some time but recently become troublesome.

Mood change of a depressive sort is a common association, obsessions get worse with depression and vice versa, so a vicious circle is set up.

Anguish, anxiety and tension are frequent accompaniments. The obsessional's tendency to self-criticism is unduly exaggerated. He or she describes symptoms in strongly self-condemnatory terms, apparently quite failing to see them as illness at all, although friends or colleagues quite easily recognize that the subject is unwell.

Differential diagnosis

The pure obsessional is often hard to distinguish from a depressive illness with obsessional features since depression usually accompanies the former. The history, however, should be helpful.

Schizophrenia may present as an obsessional illness, or obsessional features may complicate it. This can present a tricky diagnostic problem. Obsessions associated with schizophrenia tend to be rather bizarre.

Treatment

Psychotherapy

Analytic psychotherapy of obsessional illness aims at discovering the symbolic meaning of the phenomena, for the psychoanalytic view of obsessional illness is that it results from overactivity of the superego which defends the ego against overwhelming anxiety by magical rituals. In practice, obsessionals do not respond particularly well to psychotherapy; their pedantry and excessive concern with detail cause them to become enmeshed in the therapeutic process and brought to a halt. Supportive therapy, however, can help patients to ventilate pent-up feelings about their rituals and afford them some relief of anxiety and tension.

Thought stopping by reciprocal inhibition is more successful. An easy method is to ask a patient to wear an elastic band on his or her wrist and whenever the obsessional train of thought starts, to pull the band so it stings the wrist. This sounds masochistic and trite but it is very successful (and cheap!) in many milder cases.

Physical treatment

1 Drugs: clomipramine (50–200 mg per day) may be helpful in obsessional neurosis. The odd case may be helped by a monoamine-oxidase inhibitor.
2 Electroconvulsive therapy (ECT) is useful in the presence of depression.
3 Psychosurgery is used in the treatment of chronic severe obsessional disorder accompanied by persistent tension and misery.

Natural history and prognosis

Obsessional illnesses show phases of remission and exacerbation so that the long-term outlook is not so gloomy as is sometimes feared. Nevertheless the illness can be crippling. It is useful to use social criteria in assessing the degree of handicap, e.g. one should try and find out how long per day the patient spends on rituals; do they prevent him or her from working or is he or she late for work? The presence of depression of any degree makes the outlook better.

Hypochondriasis

Preoccupation with fancied bodily illness is a persistent and troublesome experience which can cause misery, prolonged and unnecessary investigation and mounting impatience in the doctor confronted with the querulous demands of the hypochondriac. For convenience it is classified with the neuroses—the majority of hypochondriacs are neurotic but at the same time it should be conceded that hypochondriasis can be delusional. The classification of hypochondrias is contentious. In general hypochondriasis may colour:

1   neurotic depression;

2   anxiety;

3   obsessional disorder; and

4   hysteria;

and bizarre hypochondriasis can occur in schizophrenia. There is a residue of hypochondriacal people who do not fit into this classification and who go through life preoccupied with their health — a history of minor ailments in childhood grossly overtreated is common. Some of these may be considered iatrogenic. Management of the hypochondriacal patient includes:

1   vigorous treatment of anxiety or depression;

2   calling a halt to unnecessary investigation;

3   individual supportive therapy by the same physician — passing the patient from one doctor to another only makes matters worse.

Finally, doctors should recognize that hypochondriasis is easily fostered in a pill-orientated age.

References

Rees, L. & Eysenck, H.J. (1945) A factorial study of some morphological and psychological aspects of human constitution. *Journal of Mental Science*, **91**, 8–21.

Schneider. K. (1958) *Psychopathic Personalities.* Cassell, London.

Slater, E. (1943) The neurotic constitution. *Journal of Neurology and Psychiatry*, **6**, 1–16.

Further reading

Beech, H. R. (1974) *Obsessional States.* Methuen, London.

Berne, E. (1984) *Games People Play.* Penguin, London.

Eysenck, H. J. (1947) *Dimensions of Personality.* Kegan Paul, London.

Freud, S. (1936) *The Problem of Anxiety,* Norton, New York.

Gaupp, R. (1974) The case of the schoolmaster Wagner. In Hirsch, S. R. & Shepherd, M. (Eds) *Themes and Variations in European Psychiatry.* John Wright, Bristol.

Guze, S. B. (1975) The validity of hysteria. *American Journal of Psychiatry*, **132**, 138–41.

Kretschmer, E. (1974) The sensitive delusion reference. In Hirsch, S. R. & Shepherd, M. (Eds) *Themes and Variations in European Psychiatry.* John Wright, Bristol.

Lewis, (1975) The survival of hysteria. *Psychological Medicine (London)*, **5**, 9–12.

Rees, L. (1950) Body size, personality and neurosis. *Journal of Mental Science*, **96**, 168.

Rotter, J. B. (1966) Generalized expectancies for internal versus external control of reinforcement. *University of Connecticut Psychological Monographs*, **80** (1), 1–28.

Sargant, W. (1957) *Battle for the Mind.* Heinemann, London.

Satir, V. (1987) *Peoplemaking.* Souvenir Press, London.

Appendix

Desensitization by paradoxical intention (DPI)

'Phobic neurosis' (ICD 300.2) is the scientific name for the condition your psychiatrist considers you are suffering from. Its main features are 'panic attacks' which are really episodes of extreme anxiety. Their origin lies in the normal physical effects of the hormone, adrenaline, made in your body. Whenever you or anyone else is frightened, some adrenaline is released into the bloodstream. Its basic effect is to prepare the body to run away from what is frightening. It may be thought of as an evolutionary hangover from the days when we had to run away from tigers, etc.

Adrenaline sends blood to those bits of the body active if you're running away and takes blood away from those bits of the body that are not used in running. All this is involuntary, it is automatic, you have no control over it. Once you are frightened, you make adrenaline and the blood is redirected to muscles ready for running away.

The blood is directed away from the mouth, stomach, gut, genitals and skin: it is directed to the leg muscles, the heart, the lungs and the head, as shown by this table:

Blood stream's change	Physical effects	Your interpretation
Away from:	*You may notice:*	*Fear of:*
Mouth	Less saliva; dry mouth	Choking
Gullet	Heartburn; 'lump in throat'	Choking
Stomach	Acid, churning stomach	Ulcers
Gut	Diarrhoea; 'butterflies'	Cancer
Skin	Goose pimpling; 'creeping flesh'; flushing; sweating	
Genitals	No arousal	Impotence
To:		
Leg muscles	'Jelly legs'	Collapse
Heart	Palpitations	Heart attack
Lungs	Gasping, smothering sensation	Suffocation
Head	Wooziness; giddiness; faintness	Brain tumour or 'going mad'

If the physical effects are not understood as a normal effect of being frightened, you may find them frightening and, for example, you may think the palpitations of an increased heart rate are a heart attack coming on. *These normal physical effects will then be frightening.* You will make adrenaline because you are frightened. The physical effects will increase. You will get more frightened, you will make more adrenaline . . . .

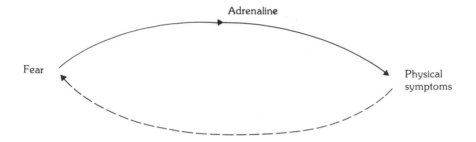

A vicious circle is set up which, when severe, is called a 'panic attack.'

To treat it, your district psychiatric nurse will ask you to provoke your fears to get the physcial symptoms. You then sit through them to learn through actual experience that nothing terrible will happen. You may know nothing terrible will happen, but emotionally you feel it will. To educate your emotions, there is no substitute for experience. This is why the nurse will ask you to provoke a 'panic'. It may seem strange at first, provoking the very thing you have been trying to avoid. But it works. If you work hard, it takes about 6 to 8 weeks to conquer your phobia.

Chapter 6
Alcoholism and Drug Dependence

Introduction

Alcoholism is a serious social problem in the UK. At least one in 20 of the population is a problem drinker. The cost is enormous; in 1987 the financial loss in industrial output through alcoholism was around £11 000 million and the cost of health and social services around £1700 million. The recognition of alcohol-related problems is now a matter of medical and social urgency of which all doctors should be aware—particularly in general practice, since too many problem drinkers pass unrecognized by too many doctors.

Definition

The term alcoholism, never easily defined, has now been replaced by alcohol-dependence and problem drinking, though the World Health Organisation retains the word alcoholism to cover dependence and problem drinking. Problem drinking is alcohol consumption which leads to physical, psychological or social problems, or all three. Alcoholics never recognize themselves as being 'alcoholics' but accept the term 'problem drinker'. Thus 'alcoholism' is retained as a term. Problem drinking should be recognized easily because it is dose related. This is something that has been clarified in recent years. The danger level is 21 units of alcohol per week for males and 14 units for females. A unit is a half pint of beer, a glass of wine or a small measure of spirits. As consumption rises the individual will develop both physical and psychological withdrawal symptoms. Physical dependence on alcohol is a dose-related syndrome in which withdrawal symptoms appear within 12 hours of the last drink. The patient sweats profusely, develops tremor, cardiac arrhythmia, retching and vomiting, and may have withdrawal fits. He or she learns to allay these symptoms by drinking.

Incidence

The incidence of alcohol-related problems is hard to estimate but the figure of one in 20 in the UK population seems definite. For this reason, early recognition of a destructive process which can destroy health, personal relationships, professional life and prospects, is very important. A conservative estimate is 2 000 000 problem drinkers in the UK. Twenty-five per cent of patients in general hospitals have alcoholic-related pathology.

Aetiology

The most important fact of aetiology is the dose level. The more alcohol a person consumes, the more damage is done. A family history of alcoholism is an important factor—alcoholics tend to have alcoholic fathers. A small percentage of alcoholics, probably less than 10%, are so-called 'symptomatic alcoholics' who are using alcohol as a form of self-medication against feelings of anxiety and/or depression, themselves made worse by the alcohol. It should be emphasized that alcoholic patients, however, are a heterogenous group of individuals damaged by a toxin. Psychological steroetypes of 'alcoholic personalities' are misleading and unhelpful. This is not to say that people do not use alcohol to relieve neurotic anxiety or escape from problems in living, in many cases they do, but social factors are highly relevant. The use of alcohol as a social lubricant in business, the tolerance of public drunkenness and heavy drinking, are all factors which encourage people not to control their drinking. Certain occupations are highly at risk, these include barmen, merchant sailors, members of the armed forces and the entertainment industry, and particularly doctors.

Clinical manifestations

Introduction

There is a pattern in the history of problem drinking which can at least aid in the diagnosis, and the following features are found to be signs that drinking is getting out of control:

1 gulping;
2 taking extra drinks before parties;
3 drinking on the way home;
4 drinking during the day;
5 lying about one's consumption of alcohol;
6 avoiding the topic of alcohol in conversation;
7 concealing alcohol on the person;
8 carrying drink to work;
9 taking liveners on rising; and
10 amnesic gaps.

The incipient alcoholic passes through a state of habitual excessive drinking bouts until he or she is drinking all the time.

The full-blown clinical picture may be easily recognized by the familiar picture of the red-faced, obese, probably bronchitic toper, moving from saloon bar joviality to maudlin tears or uncontrolled anger with easy rapidity.

Recognition and diagnosis

The recognition of the alcoholic patient consists in looking at the total picture of the patient and being on the look-out for physical complications. Often the patient presents with these and does not mention his drinking history at all. In all cases, a useful tactic is to take a complete history of the patient's drinking habits during a typical 24 hours. This is more revealing than merely asking how much the patient drinks. A raised mean corpuscular volume (MCV) and raised gamma glutamyl transferase level are excellent screening tests. Physical complications of chronic alcoholism include:

1 nausea;
2 gastritis;

3 diarrhoea;
4 hepatic cirrhosis, liver failure, portal systematic encepalopathy;
5 piles;
6 pancreatitis;
7 bronchitis;
8 pulmonary tuberculosis;
9 peripheral neuritis; peripheral neuropathy, paraparesis;
10 macrocytic anaemia;
11 hypertension and coronary heart disease;
12 late onset epilepsy; and
13 fetal alcohol syndrome (fetal damage induced by alcohol).

Psychological manifestations

Apart from the psychological changes already described there are certain complicating syndromes, namely:

Alcoholic hallucinosis

This condition is characterized by auditory hallucinations of long standing followed by the development of paranoid delusions. It is controversial whether this is a syndrome in its own right or merely the incidence of schizophrenia in an alcoholic. Typically, the onset is insidious and remits if the patient abstains from alcohol.

Delirium tremens

As the name implies, tnis is a state of restlessness and impaired consciousness associated with tremor. The onset usually follows alcoholic withdrawal and may be heralded by a 24-hour prodrome in which apprehension is prominent, and misinterpretation of the environment, mild disorientation and fits occur. The florid clinical picture reveals an excited, hallucinating (visually and aurally) patient, misinterpreting the environment in paranoid fashion and in an affective state of terror. He or she is usually restless and febrile.

Treatment consists of nursing in a bright room, the provision of plenty of fluid, vitamin saturation and the use of phenothiazine tranquillizers. These will restore normal contact with reality in under 36 hours. Chlormethiazole (Heminevrin) is a valuable antidote.

Korsakov's syndrome

This is a syndrome of gross impairment of recent memory with a tendency to confabulate answers. It was originally described in alcoholics but can also be caused by conditions such as arteriosclerosis.

Alcoholic dementia

There is nothing particular about the condition apart from the aetiology. An extremely insidious onset is the rule.

Psychosocial complications

1   Marital breakdown.
2   Loss of job.
3   General decline in personal relationships.
4   Car accidents.
5   Law breaking.
6   Aggressive behaviour and violence.

All these lead to personal catastrophe and too often end in suicide.

Treatment and prevention

The first step in treatment is withdrawal from alcohol. This can only be achieved in hospital and the successful treatment of alcoholism depends on this initial step followed by abstention. Withdrawal is not difficult to manage; it requires a degree of cooperation which reflects the patient's intention to get rid of his or her habit. And of course, the patient is under no compulsion to do this.

There is no point in prolonging the agony by giving diminishing quantities of alcohol; it is better to stop completely and be prepared to treat any complications which follow, such as fits or delirium tremens. Sedatives such as barbiturates are best avoided in the withdrawal period; most workers prefer to use chlormethiazole to allay restlessness, combined with *vitamin saturation* and plenty of fluid and nourishment. Chlormethiazole is a sedative and anticonvulsant that many regard as ideal. It can be given intravenously, e.g. in the case of associated severe illness. However, chlormethiazole itself can cause dependence so some prefer to use diazepam 20 mg every 4 hours, in reducing doses over a 6-day period.

Once the withdrawal period is over one is faced with the problem of encouraging abstention from alcohol for the rest of the patient's life. There are several ways of approaching this problem; none is complete in itself. First, by medication, disulfiram (Antabuse) provides a chemical defence against alcohol for the patient so that on taking a drink when on regular disulfiram, an unpleasant reaction occurs in which he or she feels unwell, flushes and collapses. The success of this treatment depends on the degree of cooperation that the patient is willing to offer. It is basically conditional avoidance.

The main forms of help offered to the alcoholic are psychotherapeutic and social. Individual psychotherapy probably has little to offer, but the available evidence suggests that group psychotherapy in specialized units has. It helps the alcoholic to see his or her difficulties in perspective and come to terms with the problems that drink creates, and the problems created for him or her by abstention. Not least it may outline the problems that force him or her to drink. A telling comment on this was made by a patient who said, 'It's all very well asking me to give up drinking but what are you going to put in its place?'.

Alcoholics Anonymous (AA) plays a great part in the treatment of the alcoholic and its help should be offered to all who need it. It is an organization of alcoholics devoted to helping each other to abstain from drink and has the great merit of being founded on commonsense principles of a semi-religious sort. The symptomatic alcoholic is treated by treating the underlying conditions, e.g. depression.

Modification of drinking behaviour

It is now realized that for the majority of patients total abstention is impossible to achieve and, with this in mind, current practice favours re-educating the patient in learning to return to controlled, sensible drinking. This is of course not applicable to patients who have severe associated physical damage. Such patients have to work towards total abstention. Regardless of final drinking behaviour, a period of abstention of at least 6 months is usually essential.

Prognosis

Prognosis is not precise but a few general comments can be made. The sounder the individual's personality the better the prognosis. The shorter the duration of alcoholism the better. Occupations leading to alcoholism make the prognosis worse (barmen, etc.) Patients appear to recover spontaneously after many years and the most important medical intervention maintains health pending that final recovery. Too often treatment is grudgingly or minimally provided because the chronic relapsing nature of the condition makes staff feel they are 'wasting their time'. Not so: the treatment just has to be maintained for a tediously long time.

Drug addiction

Drug addiction continues to cause medical and social concern. This started in the UK in the early 1960s with the finding of an increased incidence of self-injection with opiates, heroin particularly, by young people. As might be expected, careful examination of this phenomenon reveals that problems of drug use amongst the young were more extensive than had been realized. The whole problem should be viewed against a background of widespread consumption of psychotropic drugs in general by the population at large under medical supervision. The common drugs of dependence may be considered under three headings: stimulant, sedative and hallucinogenic drugs.

Drugs with a predominantly sedative-type action

These fall into two groups. First of all there are the sedative analgesics—in other words the opiate and opioid drugs of which the most highly prized by the user would be heroin and morphine. These are usually taken intravenously and a full-blown syndrome of addiction is characterized by the presence of physical and psychological dependence, the former being manifest by physical withdrawal symptoms if the drug is discontinued and the latter by a good deal of personal involvement with drug use. Often a person's way of life is altered so that he or she becomes very closely involved with a life style in which drug usage is the main activity. This can end up with a state of social neglect where the users spends all their time and money getting hold of drugs and neglecting themselves. There are no specific signs of dependence itself though injection marks on the arms and legs are common. The opiate abstinence syndrome includes restlessness, irritability, abdominal cramps, nausea, rhinitis and diarrhoea. Withdrawal from heroin should be carried out gradually and it is customary to use this period to improve the patient's physical state with vitamins, fluids and food. Heroin is gradually reduced and replaced by methadone by mouth. This drug has the effect of a longer duration of action and is a valuable way of treating withdrawal symptoms. Detoxification is of course only the first stage and is followed by the most difficult aspects of treatment, namely, the encouragement of abstention. Naltrexone, 50 mg mane, an opiate antagonist, can be used, rather like disulfiram for alcoholics. The euphoric effect of opiates is blocked by the naltrexone and this assists maintaining abstention. In general, encouraging patients towards abstention can be said to rest on two principles, the first of which is to try and find an alternative source of satisfaction to the use of drugs in the patient's life, and this can be done by social means where one tries to provide the patient with a different life altogether. Notable examples of this sort of manoeuvre would be the Phoenix Houses, where patients commit themselves to a drug-free life and work out their problems in vigorous open-encounter sessions. Though the relapse rate is high in opiate dependence it is unwise to take too pessimistic a view, since a great deal can be done to improve the physical and psychological status of all drug users. The second approach is to try to substitute another drug for the heroin, and current practice favours the use of methadone in this respect. Heroin itself, however, pharmaceutically pure and medically supervised, is a first step away from the degradation of illicit use.

Hypno-sedative drugs

These include barbiturates and a large number of non-barbiturate sedatives such as methaqualone. The former were often prescribed in a rather unwise fashion, producing chronic barbiturate intoxication and dependence which may arise far more frequently than may be suspected. In chronic barbiturate intoxication are found slurred speech, nystagmus and ataxia with various states of confusion. Withdrawal from barbiturates often produces fits and the withdrawal period should be treated by gradual detoxification, using pentobarbitone in divided doses reducing by 100 mg daily. It should be noted that benzodiazepines, in particular diazepam, can produce states of chronic dependency when taken in doses in excess of the normal therapeutic level and that withdrawal symptoms including withdrawal seizures and panic attacks may occur.

Stimulant drugs

The commonest in use are those of the amphetamine-type including Dexedrine, Drinamyl and Preludin. These drugs, taken by people of normal and abnormal personality for their stimulant effect, produce a short-lived feeling of well-being followed by gloom, inducing the taker to consume larger quantities of the drugs so that up to 2 g per 24 hours may be consumed.

States of *restlessness* and *irritability* with outbursts of anger are common but probably the most serious manifestation is *amphetamine psychosis* (Connell, 1958). This is a syndrome of restlessness, elation, paranoid ideas and hallucinosis, i.e. a schizophreniform psychosis, which clears up on withdrawal.

The treatment of amphetamine dependence is made more difficult by its prevalence amongst psychopaths and also by its unwise prescription. It should be emphasized that there are really only three clear indications for the use of amphetamines: in narcolepsy, in over-sedated epileptic patients, and in the treatment of hyperkinetic children.

In recent years, cocaine has become a widely used stimulant taken by inhalation. It is a euphoriant as well as a stimulant and this accounts for its popularity. Regular excessive use can produce reversible psychosis with characteristic tactile hallucinations. Serious side-effects are necrotic lesions in the lungs or nose due to vasoconstriction.

Hallucinogenic drugs

Hallucinogenic drugs have been more widely used in recent years since the early 1960s. The most commonly misused of these is the diethylamide salt of lysergic acid (LSD) and although it does not produce any physical dependence it can certainly cause states of psychological dependence where the individual overvalues its supposed effects on his mental state. In unhappy individuals, or when taken in states of anxiety, lysergide is associated with adverse reactions and in general these tend to fall into three types: states of acute psychotic excitment, depressive states, and states of panic and terror, often followed by persistent symptoms of depersonalization. Fortunately the majority of adverse lysergide reactions appear to subside spontaneously, though ideally such patients should receive psychiatric supervision and admission when necessary.

Other hallucinogenic drugs which may be encountered include the following:

1 *Phencyclidine* which is becoming a fairly widely used 'street drug'.

2 *Psilocybin* in the form of 'magic mushrooms' (liberty caps) which grow commonly throughout England. Between ten and 30 caps are boiled to make a tea. The effects are similar to lysergide but less intense. They are responsible for the autumn appearance in casualty departments of alarmed, disorientated youths. Spontaneous recovery, with or without symptomatic sedation, is the rule.

3 *Indian hemp from Cannabis species*, especially *C. indica*, is available chiefly as the grassy stems (marijuana) or the resinous exudate of the flowers (hashish). In susceptible individuals, e.g. schizophrenics, symptoms are aggravated and symptomatic treatment is helpful.

Aetiology

Botany provides a useful analogy for the aetiology of addiction to alcohol or any other substance: Consider the *drug* as the *seed*, each having its differing properties; consider the *addict* as the *soil* in which the seed lands, different people have differing propensities to addiction (see, for example, Rotter's 'locus of control', p. 10). Consider the cultural environment or *society* in which that individual is brought up as the *climate*.

Though the seed and the soil are important, the climate is overwhelmingly so. The contrast between the Amazon jungle and the Sahara desert well demonstrate this. Alcoholism is rare in Arabia, common in Scotland. Curiously, however, prohibition in free, secular societies like England appear to be associated with increases in demand and consumption: American domestic heroin consumption has risen every year, year on year, since 1923 *when the drug was prohibited*. With no restraints, such as in the London of Hogarth's days, consumption also rose, so that prohibition and free availability both appear to lead to excessive problematic use. Only a happy medium of *controlled availability* controls (and minimizes) drug use.

Better understanding of the pharmacology of drug dependence has been achieved by the identification of drug receptors, in particular, opiate receptors in the brain and central nervous system. In addition, the identification of naturally occurring pentapeptides in the brain—the encephalins—which have opiate-like properties, leads to the hypothesis that chronic opiate abuse would suppress the activity of encephalins, thus accounting for the onset of withdrawal symptoms when the drug is discontinued.

People rarely become dependent on drugs by accident; for example, severe therapeutic dependence remains uncommon. It should be remembered that dependency-producing drugs are in general 'mind altering', i.e. they may affect feeling, perception, thinking and behaviour. Also, the potential user will have heard about the supposed effects and wants to try them out. This means that dependence may follow a repeated, pleasant, drug-induced effect or follow the use of a drug which abolishes some unplesant subjective symptoms, in some cases neurotic anxiety, for example, so that the drug becomes a form of self-medication.

The terms 'hard' and 'soft' drugs are misleading. A more useful distinction may be drawn between those who inject themselves with drugs and those who swallow them. The former group are more likely to develop severe varieties of dependence fairly quickly, and they also have an associated morbidity and mortality from the effects of unsterile self-injection.

Society is presently most concerned about hedonic drug use amongst young males. But these patients, though they present urgent social problems, should not deflect interest in the wider problems of 'hidden' dependency on sedatives, hypnotics and tranquillizers.

A useful way of regarding drug dependence is to realize that it often involves 'drug-using behaviour', i.e. a life style, rather than mere pharmacological dependence. At present youthful drug dependence is notable for subcultural drug use, and attitudes and a view of the world that may go with it. Multiple drug use is becoming more common.

Drug dependence, though it may ostensibly be related to such ephemera as 'curiosity' or 'a new experience' is in severe cases an outgrowth of long-standing personality disorder, often of psychopathic dimensions, but this *does not account for all cases*. Some may use drugs to relieve anxiety and depression or as a barrier between themselves and a world which they find unacceptable. For the deliquent youngster drugs may provide an easy source of illicit gratification.

Drugs come and go. Thirty years ago cocaine use had virtually disappeared. At present it has reached epidemic proportions in the USA. The same may be said of the spread of inhalation of volatile solvents in certain parts of the UK. It may, however, be worth bearing in mind that no society in history has been without its psychotropic drug. Recognition of this human foible may go a long way to putting the various drug-taking peccadilloes into perspective. For example, the emotional over-reaction to the misuse of opium and the sublime indifference to the widespread damage wrought by alcohol are arbitrary in the extreme.

Reference

Connell, P. (1958) *Amphetamine Psychosis*. Chapman & Hall, London and Maudsley Monograph No. 5, Oxford University Press, London.

Further reading

Ashton, H. (1974) Benzodiazepine withdrawal. *British Medical Journal*, **288**, 1135–40.
Berridge, V. (1987) *Opium and the People*. Yale University Press, New Haven.
Dorn, N. & South, N. (1987) *A Land fit for Heroin?* Macmillan, London.
Edwards, G. (Ed.) (1987) *Drug Scenes*. Royal College of Psychiatrists, London.
Glatt, M. M. (1983) *Alcohol, our Favourite Drug*. Royal College of Psychiatrists, London.
Kessel, W. & Walton, H. (1979) *Alcoholism*. Penguin, London.
Maier, H. W. (1987) *Cocainism*. Addiction Research Foundation, Toronto.
Stewart, T. (1987) *The Heroin Users*. Pandora, London.
Zinberg, N. E. (1984) *Drugs Set and Setting*. Yale University Press, New Haven.

Chapter 7
Psychosexual Disorders

Introduction

It is only in the last few years that any reference to psychosexual disorders has had a place in the undergraduate medical curriculum. This was an amazing gap in the training of doctors since it left them with very limited understanding of common sexual problems and meant that they were unable to offer advice or help in many cases. This was probably backed up by a hangover from more prudish attitudes of the past when the discussion of sexual matters at any level was practically taboo. There were of course a number of physicians and psychiatrists who had the interest and ability to deal with the problems of patients with psychosexual disorders, but they were relatively few and the literature was sparse. Above and beyond this there was little experimental work to back up many of the pronouncements on psychosexual topics which were made mainly on the basis of untested theories, often highly speculative. However, in more recent times, starting with the work of Kinsey on the varieties of sexual practice in the American population and more recently with the experimental work of Masters and Johnston on the treatment of common psychosexual disorders, the topic has at last found its place in undergraduate medical teaching. We may add to this the fact that public demand for help with their sexual problems naturally became greater as the public became aware through the media that research and active therapy was available in various parts of the world, notably the USA.

Patients with sexual problems undergo a great deal of unhappiness and misery and if help is not available it can lead to marital breakdown, depressive states, alcohol abuse, drug abuse and suicidal attempts. Clearly the management of psychosexual disorders is not entirely the province of the physician, in fact contemporary approaches to these problems involves a multidisciplinary approach in which physicians, psychiatrists, psychologist and social workers will all make their relevant contributions. But the doctor is frequently the first person consulted, and there are recognizable groups of common psychosexual problems that every doctor should know about. The most common psychosexual problems include:

1 erectile failure, i.e. impotence in the male;
2 premature ejaculation; and
3 failure to achieve orgasm in the female. This term is preferable to 'frigidity', an unhappy term which should be dropped.

Erectile failure

Erectile failure is simply related to anxiety based on fear of loss of sexual potency, and this can arise in various ways; probably the commonest are ignorance, inexperience or long-standing fears about potency which may go well back into puberty. Another common cause is failure to achieve erection at the first attempt at sexual intercourse.

This sort of erectile failure may convince the man that he is incapable of achieving erection, and repeated failures reinforce the condition, leaving the patient with the belief that the disorder is quite untreatable. Approximately 90% of cases of erectile failure arise out of anxiety, but there are obviously important physical causes including neurological disorders such as diabetic neuropathy and spinal cord lesions and also it may be found in patients whose general physical health is below par, e.g. through chronic cardiac disorders. Endocrine causes of erectile failure are actually relatively rare but obviously need to be borne in mind. It should be remembered that there are many drugs that will contribute to erectile failure, including any hypno-sedative or tranquillizer taken regularly; perhaps the commonest of these is alcohol in excess, and certainly all the tricyclic antidepressants produce erectile failure as a side-effect. It is also found in patients who are taking antihypertensive medications. Heavy smokers are at risk too.

Treatment

A full and detailed history of the patient's sexual development, range of experience and attitudes towards sexuality is a prerequisite. Most healthy males experience spontaneous early morning erections, probably due to recruited stimulation by a full bladder. Impotence due to psychological factors such as anxiety does not affect early morning erection, but all erections are banished by physical damage such as neuropathy.

Having excluded physical or pharmacological causes, one is left in the vast majority of cases with a patient whose failure is related to anxiety. The impotent patient cannot be treated on his own. It is important always to secure the cooperation of the sexual partner and go very carefully into all the details of the development of the patient's impotence. Having established the extent of the problem, the usual recommendation is to advise partners to abstain from sexual intercourse. The value of this is that it helps both the patient and the partner to have a cooling off period where the resentment, ill-feeling and general wretchedness that have usually built up can be allowed to subside. It is also important to make it clear to both that this is a treatable condition, with the doctor positive, supportive and encouraging in attitude.

Space does not permit a detailed examination of the various therapeutic techniques involved, but the principles can be summarized by saying that the first essential is to clarify the history from the point of view of both partners as fully as possible, to advise a period of abstention for several weeks and then to commence upon therapy. The general principles of therapy now employed tend to involve the patient in a process of re-education so that sexual activity is approached without anxiety and the partner is advised not to react in a rejecting and unhappy way if erection is not achieved but gradually to build up sexual activity without aiming at complete penetration. The idea then is to rehabilitate the lost sexual function in a non-stressful way; thus by gaining confidence, the patient's erections will return to normal and satisfactory sexual intercourse will then follow. Prognosis is notoriously difficult but there does now seem to be a consensus of opinion that if a man has been impotent for a period in excess of 2 years then success rates are extremely low; below 2 years success rates may be as high as 80% or more.

Premature ejaculation

Premature ejaculation is extremely common, and again causes great unhappiness and bitterness on the part of the disappointed sexual partner; but it is probably the most treatable of psychosexual disorders, provided the full cooperation of the partner is available. Contemporary mainstay of therapy is to advise the partner to compress the glans penis firmly just before ejaculation and this will inhibit it. If this is followed by a period of rest, intercourse may be recommenced and ejaculation delayed. It is merely a question of practice.

Failure of female orgasm

This is probably one of the unhappiest areas of psychosexual dysfunction. For many years it was claimed that the female orgasm was caused by vaginal stimulation by the erect penis and many women found themselves labelled as frigid because this did not seem to occur. In fact, they felt cheated, disappointed and often felt themselves less than fully female because they had not achieved this widely described experience. However, experimental evidence has shown that in fact female orgasm is mainly caused by clitoral stimulation and that the vaginal orgasm is relatively rare. Again, with good cooperation between sexual partners and advice about clitoral stimulation, manual, oral and for that matter mechanical, most women who may have been labelled 'frigid' for years are able to achieve satisfactory orgasm and happy sexual relations which they felt had previously been denied to them.

Sexual deviations

Here we face problems of definition; in the past male and female homosexuality were considered to be sexually pathological, but the present view is that this is not the case and that male and female homosexuals are merely deviants, so that attempts to change a person's sexual orientation from homosexual to heterosexual is now rarely attempted except in those cases where the patient particularly requests it.

At the same time it has to be remembered that homosexuals of either sex are often the victims of a good deal of persecution by society that regards their sexual lives as immoral and disgusting. This can lead to a great deal of unhappiness, particularly in young male homosexuals who can become severely depressed and make suicidal attempts. Homosexuals therefore are perhaps more vulnerable to mood disturbance, guilty feelings, etc. than otherwise, and will need sympathetic and straightforward counselling in order to help them to live with themselves. Public attitudes have softened to a certain extent, and for that matter, homosexual acts between male consenting adults are no longer against the law, but this has not removed from the homosexual a considerable amount of unhappiness and vulnerability.

It is important to recognize the distinction between homosexual orientation, that is a person whose sexual preference is entirely for the same sex, and homosexual behaviour. By homosexual behaviour we refer to homosexual acts which occur in highly specialized situations, in other words in one-sex communities where no heterosexual outlet is available. Another point that needs sympathetic care encompasses the problem that many young adolescents may have regarding their sexual identity: they may have doubts as to whether or not they are homosexual or heterosexual. Sensible psychotherapy will usually help them to solve this problem. Male homosexuals may be primary (trans-sexual) or secondary (fetishistic).

Fetishism

This is usually regarded as a sexual deviation and implies that condition where the person may only achieve orgasm after being stimulated by various inanimate objects ranging from shoes or black rubber raincoats to even more bizarre outfits. The male of the species particularly readily imprints, i.e. forms conditional stimuli. Rubber fetishists may relate to the fact that many males' first sexual experience involves the use of a rubber condom. Boys with a normal heterosexual development may experience their first sexual act with an older homosexual. By imprinting they then become 'facultative' or secondary homosexuals.

Sadism and masochism

These are a pathological exaggeration of the sexual relationship and are on the whole to be regarded as serious and often dangerous sexual deviations since they include enjoyment of pain (masochism) or of the infliction of pain (sadism) as a sexual preamble to orgasm. It will be wise always to refer such patients who ask for help to a psychiatrist.

Transvestism

Transvestism, often called cross-dressing, merely means the drive, usually in the male, to dress up in female clothing, either as a way of obtaining sexual relief or before having heterosexual intercourse. It is not, as is often supposed, a homosexual behaviour. Indeed, over-sexed males may be excited by the surrogate contact with female genitals that mere contact with female underwear offers. It would be difficult to say whether this is a state that needs treating: probably the most important criterion is whether it makes the transvestite or his sexual partner unhappy.

Trans-sexualism

This means the desire to change sex. This is an entirely different area from transvestism and is mainly seen in men who wish to become female. It is thought to arise from early in utero exposure of the brain of a male fetus to inappropriate levels of circulating maternal adrenalin, or other hormones. Although genotypically male, social and even hormonal responses may be female. The patient may express the conviction that 'from early childhood I felt I was a woman trapped in a man's body'. This 'primary homosexuality' is also known in females who desire plastic construction of a penis, but this is very rare. Trans-sexuals are often extremely determined in this respect and males will undergo extensive surgery, penile amputation and the creation of an artificial vagina, breast implants and so on. Psychiatry has had little success in persuading them to change their attitudes. Phenothiazines may help. The really determined trans-sexual will attain his goal if at all possible, using threats of suicide as persuasion.

Limited experience suggests that too often trans-sexualism overlies quite deep-seated personality problems even to the extent of serious personality disorder. The ethics of surgical sex transformation are in the authors' opinions highly questionable.

Rape

Much has been made of the sadistic urge of the male and the masochistic urge of the female that is claimed by some to be essential for true sexual passion. What is undoubted is that this can be excessive and, in the male, lead to assault of the opposite sex. The causes may be hormonal, treatable with cyproterone, or psychological, such as an inferiority complex that makes a man unable to approach women until a build up of libidinous drive leads to a pathological outlet of excessive, sometimes sadistic behaviour. Treatment of these problems is difficult and controversial and ranges from demands for punitive terms of imprisonment or castration to lobbying by prostitutes' organizations for recognition of their therapeutic role. The appropriate remedy is to pinpoint the reasons for what is, first and foremost, an assault and violation of the liberty of another individual. Only if this elementary insight and recognition of the equality of others is gained will treatment of hormonal disorder or pathological personality be lastingly successful.

Further reading

Berne, E. (1986) Sex in Human Loving. Penguin, London.
Kaplan, H. (1974) Sex Therapy. Ballière Tindall, London.
Parker, T. (1970) The Twisting Lane. Panther, London.
Sevely, J. L. (1987) Eve's Secrets. Bloomsbury, London.
Storr, A. (1972) Sexual Deviation. Pelican, London.
West, D. J. (1972) Homosexuality. Pelican, London.

Chapter 8
Mental Handicap

Introduction

The public often confuses the distinction between mental illness and mental handicap. This is made worse by the many changes of terminology that have taken place. It is important to make the effort to use the current terminology, because people with a mental handicap (and their families and service providers) are sometimes sensitive about the labels that are applied.

The disability underlying mental handicap is a *learning difficulty*, that is, an impairment of intelligence. The term is only used for handicaps that are established during the developmental period (i.e. before school-leaving age). The key features of mental handicap are *impaired social adaptation* due to *intellectual impairment* arising during *development*.

By way of contrast, the key features of a mental illness are:

1 it is *acquired*, identifiable as a change of functioning:
2 the change involves *impaired psychological* (not necessarily intellectual) *functioning*; and
3 these impairments form a recognizable pattern or *syndrome*.

Impairment of intelligence commencing after school-leaving is mental illness (dementia), not mental handicap. Any illness (including mental illness), arising before school-leaving age, which leads to permanent intellectual impairment, may be a cause of mental handicap.

Whose handicap?

Because handicap is defined socially, it is important to recognize that a given level of disability is associated with a wide range of social adaptation. Someone with mild learning difficulties may have a job, marry, raise children, and never require professional services; or else may require daily support, with residential and day services. The difference is due to the social environment and its effect on education and personality development. Figure 6 shows an individual within a family, in contact with specialist services and general services, all embedded in society. These are the sources of handicap for each.

For the individual

1 Primary disability includes impaired learning of the skills required for independent living, communication skills, social skills and strategies for coping with stress (including illness).
2 Secondary disability includes lack of positive social roles, which leads to lack of sense of identity, lack of relationships, low self-esteem, lack of fulfilment and frustration.
3 Tertiary disability (i.e. reaction to other people's attitudes) includes

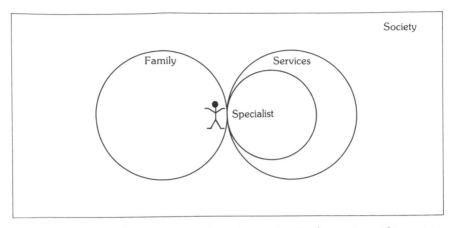

Fig. 6 Venn diagram showing a mentally handicapped patient's situation within society.

acquiescence, suggestibility, excessive shyness, and some behaviour that is inappropriate to the person's age or the social context.

For the family

1   Psychological responses include immediate emotional reactions (described as similar to grief), long-term reactions, adaptive or maladaptive coping responses. Extremes such as rejection or denial of disability are rare, but psychologically very damaging.

2   Social effects include financial cost, time, the prospect of permanent dependency, and loss of opportunities for employment, leisure and relationships. The recognition of handicap presents a crisis for many marriages; the rate of separation is high in the first few years, but thereafter is low.

3   The effects on health, surprisingly, appear to be minimal.

For specialist services

Working in a mental handicap service is sometimes stressful, and has low status. There is a vicious circle of chronic underfunding, poor training, staff 'burnout', high turnover of staff, and difficulties in recruiting high-quality staff. This is linked to the fact that such services are traditionally segregated from services for the rest of the population, even where they serve the same purpose (e.g. schools).

For general services

People with a mental handicap form a small proportion of the clientele of any general service, such as the health service. Extra effort is required to take account of their individual needs. For example, someone might be unable to sit patiently in a waiting room, and may need to have the first appointment of a session. The problems of communication may be daunting, and the effort may not seem worthwhile.

For society

Society places a high value on skill, knowledge, conformity to social norms, and the fulfilment of roles (such as parent, friend, employee, etc.). People who do not have these characteristics are devalued, and fill deviant roles. The names used for such people become insults, and various stereotyped caricatures are used to describe them. Common stereotypes include 'the eternal child' and 'the buffoon'. People viewed as deviant become targets for ridicule, exploitation, deprivation, crime and cruelty.

Terminology

At one time, little distinction was made between mental handicap and mental illness, but gradually 'born fools' were distinguished from 'lunatics'. The terms 'idiot', 'imbecile' and 'moron' were widely used (e.g. by Shakespeare), but given a technical definition in the 1917 Mental Deficiency Act. They were removed from official language by the 1959 Mental Health Act, which introduced 'mental subnormality'. This was supposed to refer to the statistical concept of performance less than two standard deviations below the mean on an intelligence test. The term was rarely used so precisely, and was unpopular with families because it had connotations of 'subhuman'. It was abolished by the 1983 Mental Health Act, which introduced the term 'mental impairment'. This has a precise legal definition, and refers to a small subset of people with a mental handicap, so it should not be used as a synonym. The definition is 'a state of arrested or incomplete development of mind, including significant impairment of intelligence and social functioning, and associated with abnormally aggressive or seriously irresponsible conduct on the part of the person concerned'.

The term used in most other countries, by the World Health Organisation and in the scientific literature is 'mental retardation'. The term is unpopular with families in this country, who prefer 'mental handicap' at present. Each term is introduced in an attempt to reduce the pejorative connotations of its predecessor; but the further the word is from ordinary English, the worse an insult it becomes. For example, to be called a 'spastic' in the school playground is considered worse than being called a 'fool'. When speaking to families, avoid technical terms which they have only heard as insults. The most descriptive English words which cause least offence are 'slow', 'slow learner', and perhaps 'backward'.

There is no advantage in using a collective term to describe people with mental handicaps. Diversity and individuality are the common factors. It is much preferable to refer to people in terms of the roles they are fulfilling. At school, the person is a pupil; in the family, a son, sister, etc; in other contexts, a tenant, a customer, a friend; and in a doctor's surgery, a patient.

Assessment

Ordinary medical history-taking is not appropriate for assessing permanent disabilities. However, a mentally handicapped person will usually be consulting a doctor about an illness, and details of that illness should be recorded first. Include a heading 'pre-morbid level of function' after recording 'pre-morbid

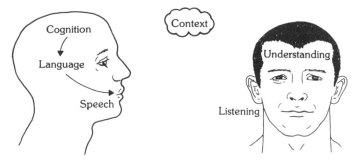

Fig. 7 The main components of communication.

personality'. This should be an account of a 'typical day' from rising, washing, choosing clothes, dressing, etc., through getting to work, and so on to using leisure time and getting ready for bed. One should record how much the person can do if encouraged, rather than what they habitually do.

There are many standardized forms of assessment. IQ tests such as the Wechsler Adult Intelligence Scale (WAIS) have restricted uses including epidemiology, assessment of specific intellectual functions, and determining, whether someone's handicaps are due to intellectual impairment; they are also useful in adult-onset disorders, to find out whether they are stable or progressive.

IQ tests do not help you to answer questions like 'What can this person do for himself?' and 'How much assistance is needed?' What skills is he ready to learn? There are now many assessments available such as Pathways to Independence, or the American Adaptive Behaviour Scale.

Specialized tests have to be used by trained people, usually psychologists. 'Pathways' does not require training. It is worth obtaining a copy of the adaptive behaviour assessment used by the mental handicap service in the locality. Some psychologists are reluctant to use IQ tests because they have been misused in the past. The WAIS should be regarded as a sharp tool like a chisel, not to be used as a screwdriver.

The main task for a doctor is to take a history, and the problem is, how to communicate. Problems may originate in any of the spheres shown in Fig. 7 and described below.

1 Cognition The person may not have the intention to communicate, or form the ideas he or she wishes to convey. He or she may not have clear or accurate concepts of time.

2 Language ability. The patient may not have the vocabulary to express symptoms, nor be able to find the right word. He or she may have difficulty with using the correct syntax, pronunciation, etc. He or she may have pragmatic deficits, e.g. difficulty with making appropriate eye contact, or in replying relevantly to questions.

3 Speech production. The patient may have difficulty with the pitch, articulation, intonation, rhythm, rate or volume of speech.

4 *Listening*. The patient may have difficulty keeping his or her attention on the interview.

5 *Understanding*. He or she may not understand the doctor's vocabulary, the meaning of complex concepts (e.g. 'mood') or the complexity of the doctor's syntax.

6 *Context*. He or she may not understand the purpose and context of the interview, the role of a doctor or the rules of confidentiality. There are some very specific social skills required by patients when consulting doctors, e.g. how to obtain an appointment.

Furthermore, motor and sensory impairments are more common, so you should always check if the person uses a hearing aid (and if it is switched on), and sit with your face and lips well lit.

To deal with these dificulties requires systematic application of ordinary interview techniques:

1 Assess the person's ability to communicate. The first few minutes of a medical interview are not simply 'to establish rapport', but should be used for this purpose. Even a very severely handicapped person will reply to 'What is your name?'. With practice, one can judge what level of complexity of questioning each patient understands.

2 Be systematic. If there is a communication problem, work out which components of communication are affected and how you would interview a patient who *only* had that problem, and then combine those techniques. For example, a foreigner taught English at school might be deficient only in vocabulary. One would use gesture, pictures, offer alternative words which might be recognized, speak slowly and clearly, restrict the range of vocabulary used, and use an interpreter. Work out for yourself what kind of patient might have an isolated defect of another aspect of communication.

3 There are three ways to use a third party. You may need someone as an *informant*, but tell them that you would like to find out how much the person can tell you on their own, and that you will check details with them. Sometimes an *interpreter* is useful, to help you understand the patient's language and vice versa. Sometimes the patient could give a better history if taught how to do so, and you could ask someone (such as a mental handicap nurse) to act as an *instructor*. For example, the patient could be taught how to keep a diary of sleep problems.

4 Rehearse your questions. Throughout your career you will be asking patients the same questions. Listen to yourself, preferably by tape recording some real interviews. How could you simplify the language of your routine questions? Journalists on tabloid newspapers are highly paid because of their skill in communicating. Copy their methods but not their subject matter.

5 Hold several short interviews rather than one long one. An unfamiliar situation makes it harder to understand any communication that takes place, so your patients will understand you better if they are familiar with you and your office. Fatigue also impairs communication. Repeat interviews give you opportunities for serial observations.

6 Use other sources of information, such as school records, school medical records and social work records.

Other developmental disorders

Phrases like 'learning difficulty', 'intellectual impairment' and 'mental handicap' are sometimes used interchangeably, but learning difficulties leading to handicap in adulthood may result from a variety of developmental disorders, such as:

1 specific learning difficulties, e.g. aphasia;
2 autism (and related conditions);
3 hyperkinetic syndrome; and
4 personality disorders.

It is important to identify these disorders as soon as possible, so that appropriate teaching at school can be provided. For example, people with aphasia may benefit from an enriched language programme, possibly including the use of sign language. People with autism may need an approach that uses non-social rewards to encourage learning.

Autism is a rare condition (occurring in about 4 : 10 000 people). The features are: impaired social interaction, impaired language development, odd responses to the environment (especially the social environment) and impaired imagination. Typical 'odd' responses include resistance to any changes, and attachments to objects. Some individuals have unimpaired abilities in non-social areas such as mathematics, music or drawing; and a few individuals are talented. One-third of adolescents with autism develop epilepsy.

Hyperkinetic syndrome is also rare, and the features are impaired attention, impulsivity and restless overactvity. The hyperkinesis is often conspicuous in childhood, but sometimes gives way to underactivity in adulthood. The impairments of switching attention and filtering out unwanted stimuli are persistent, so it is sometimes called 'attention deficit disorder'.

Both these disorders are usually (but not always) associated with intellectual impairment, are commoner in males, are strongly associated with other signs of brain dysfunction, and frequently lead to behavioural problems. Consequently, they come to the attention of doctors more often than most forms of mental handicap. Services for adults with these disorders are provided by mental handicap services.

Personality disorders are common in the general population, and are only occasionally the sole cause of mental handicap. Although education takes place in the context of a relationship between a teacher and child, even children with severe relationship problems learn enough to look after themselves practically, if not emotionally. It used to be thought that personality disorder was an invariable component of mental handicap, because it is so common in people with intellectual impairments.

Some other disorders may be developmentally determined (e.g. eating disorders, sexual disorders), but they are unlikely to cause schooling problems, and do not lead to mental handicap.

Epidemiology

There are methodological problems in measuring the prevalence of mental handicap:

1 the definition is imprecise;

2   the definition depends on the social context;
3   there is no clear cut-off point between handicap and non-handicap.

For example, the prevalence found by measuring performance on IQ tests is different from that found by assessing social competence; and competence at school is very different from competence in a doctor's surgery.

In practice, the most reliable surveys have been done using IQ tests with secondary school pupils. IQ tests are scored using an assumption that the frequency distribution is Gaussian, being adjusted so that the mean = 100, and the standard deviation = 15. Although there is a 'borderline' around IQ 70, most people with a lower score (70–85) would be regarded as mentally handicapped, and most with a higher score would not.

If the Gaussian assumption were accurate, the frequency of IQ less than 70 should be 2.5%. Surveys have given widely differing estimates around that figure. However, the prevalence of 'severe mental handicap' (IQ less than 50) is much more robust between surveys in this country and abroad, and at different times. The figure is 0.3%–0.4%. This means that a GP with a list of 2000 patients might expect to have three children and five adults with a severe mental handicap on the list.

Measuring the incidence is even more difficult, because detection of handicap does not take place at the same age for everyone. Studies have been carried out on Down's syndrome because it is recognizable at birth, and nearly always causes severe mental handicap. They show that the incidence has fallen because fewer women have babies after their mid-thirties. The level in England in the late 1970s was estimated at between 0.65 and 1.06 per thousand live births. Improved life expectancy means that the prevalence may be increasing.

Aetiology

There are too many syndromes that can cause mental handicap to commit to memory. Even psychiatrists specializing in mental handicap only see a small proportion. What is required is an approach to investigating the aetiology of handicap of any particular patient seen. Details of the medically important and the commonest syndromes should be learned from a paediatric text. These include Down's syndrome, fragile-X syndrome, phenylketonuria, hypothyroidism and a few others. The frequency of some causes (e.g. malnutrition, birth trauma) differ between countries, and figures given here apply to Western Europe.

Beware of the popular myths, 'birth trauma' and 'vaccine damage'. Head injury at the time of birth is extremely rare, and it remains controversial whether pertussis vaccine can cause encephalitis.

Causes are usually classified according to the time they operate: pre-natal, peri-natal, post-natal and unknown. The proportions from a recent Swedish study are shown in Table 2.

In this study, 29% of cases of SMH were caused by chromosomal disorders, largely trisomy 21, the commonest single cause. Single gene defects accounted for 5% of SMH. Disorders acquired *in utero* include fetal alcohol syndrome (8% of MMH, but 0% of SMH in this study), diagnostic X-radiation, infection (use the

Table 2 Proportional incidence of mental handicap at various stages of life

Time	Proportion of SMH (%)	Proportion of MMH (%)
Pre-natal	55	23
Peri-natal	15	18
Post-natal	11	2
Unknown	18	55

SMH = severe mental handicap; MMH = mild mental handicap.

mnemonic ToRCHeS = toxoplasmosis, rubella, cytomegalovirus, herpes, syphilis), drugs (especially anticonvulsants), and maternal phenylketonuria.

Prenatal causes overlap with perinatal ones, which are mostly due to placental insufficiency, asphyxia and hypoxia. When a 'small-for-dates' baby is born, it may be difficult to establish when the problem started.

Postnatal causes include the whole range of diseases affecting the brain in childhood. These include trauma (accidental and non-accidental), toxic (drugs and heavy metals), metabolic (e.g. hypernatraemia due to incorrectly formulated milk), infection (meningitis and encephalitis) and malnutrition.

Mental handicap and health

People of all ages with a mental handicap face an increased risk of illness, and overall their life expectancy is reduced. However, life expectancy has been increasing rapidly in the past 30 years. It is clear that the main factor has been the change in the social and environmental conditions in which people live.

There are some health problems that are specifically associated with certain causes of handicap, there are some that are non-specific associations which share a common aetiology, and other conditions to which all mentally handicapped people have an increased susceptibility.

1   *Specific associations.* As there are so many handicapping conditions, it is impossible to list all associations here. Down's syndrome is associated with congenital cardiac defects, hypothyroidism, obesity, problems associated with viscous secretions (recurrent chest infections, acne, glue ear and conductive deafness), and early onset of syndromes normally associated with age (chronic leukaemia, Alzheimer's disease).

2   *Shared aetiology.* Any disorder affecting brain function in childhood may cause mental handicap, and may produce other phenomena of brain dysfunction. Epilepsy is 10–20 times commoner in people with severe mental handicap. Autism and hyperkinetic syndrome are strongly associated with intellectual impairment, as well as with other neurological signs.

Sensory and motor impairments (cerebral palsy) are common. Both will cause communication problems which may exacerbate the learning difficulties. The speech of individuals with severe cerebral palsy may be incomprehensible to strangers, even though they may have no intellectual impairment, so they require careful assessment. As an example of shared aetiology, rubella syndrome may cause profound deafness, blindness and intellectual impairment. 3 *Increased susceptibility.* The most important category is mental illness, which is about twice as common in people with a mental handicap as in the general population. There are great difficulties in determining accurate numbers, but it seems that schizophrenia is twice as common, manic-depressive illness is equally common, psychiatric complications of epilepsy are commoner, personality and behavioural disorders are frequent, especially if there are developmental disorders such as autism, Pre-senile dementia due to Alzheimer's disease associated with Down's syndrome is expected to be an increasing problem. Other general susceptibilities are attributable to the consequences of poor social and health care, such as TB and hepatitis B.

Mental handicap services

Most mentally handicapped people are not ill for most of the time. Handicapping conditions in childhood may require medical treatment, but by adulthood the majority of conditions have become stable. The role of a doctor is to deal with illnesses, treating the mentally handicapped patient in the same way as the rest of the population. When ill, a mentally handicapped person is entitled to expect the same standard of health care that is offered to everyone else. A mild additional illness might make the difference between somebody being able to cope and failing to do so. It may cost the family and the community more than if the same illness affected a non-handicapped person. It is not only required ethically, but is usually cost-effective, to ensure that his or her illnesses are thoroughly investigated and treated.

For historical reasons, psychiatry is the only speciality which has consultant posts wholly devoted to mental handicap, although many paediatricians have developed a special interest. There are some doctors in community health whose job is to conduct health surveillance programmes, offer advice on contraception, etc. Regrettably few neurologists take an interest, despite the frequency of neurological disorders.

Non-medical services are provided by the NHS, local authority social services, education authorities and voluntary and private agencies. The pattern varies widely around the country, and the situation is changing rapidly. To generalize, most parts of the country aim to provide local services based on Community Mental Handicap Teams (CMHTs). These carry out assessments, plan programmes of training and care (based on individual strengths and needs), implement such plans and review progress, and provide family support. The aim is progressively to increase the extent to which their clients lead valued lives by participating in the ordinary life of the community.

Membership of a CMHT often comprises a 'core' team of a social worker and a community mental handicap nurse, with secretarial support, and a 'peripheral' team of psychologist, occupational therapist, physiotherapist, speech therapist, psychiatrist, and possibly others. The peripheral staff may work with more than one core team in a district.

Day services include education, training, employment, recreation and leisure. Since the early 1970s all children have been obliged to attend school, and most education authorities have provided special schools. Since the early 1980s, mentally handicapped children have been entitled to remain in full-time education until they are 19 years old. Some colleges of further education provide suitable courses for handicapped adults. Other services are mostly provided by the NHS from mental handicap hospitals and by social services from day centres. There are a few schemes which are finding sheltered employment, and a few focusing on leisure.

Residential services include short-term care and permanent accommodation. These could be provided in a range of settings: placement with another family, provision of staff in the family home to help out, communal homes (hostels and hospitals), shared houses ('group homes'). Some mentally handicapped people live alone in their own home. Depending on the person's ability, emotional needs and behaviour, more or less staffing may be needed in any of these settings: from weekly visits to part-time and full-time staff.

Further reading

Bicknell, J. & Sines, D. (1984) *The Mentally Handicapped Person in the Community*. Harper & Row, London.

Heaton-Ward, W. A. (1977) *Left Behind*. Macdonald & Evans, Plymouth.

Russell, O. (1985) *Mental Handicap*. Churchill Livingstone, Edinburgh.

Chapter 9
Disorders of Childhood and Adolescence

Introduction

Child psychiatry is unlike adult psychiatry in that the patient is brought along by his or her parents and does not present him or herself with the problem or complaint. The presenting symptoms is seen by the parents as the problem but often the symptom can be construed as resulting from the family patterns of interaction, the parents' style of parenting or the unfortunate predicaments in which some children may find themselves. It is essential that a full and detailed history is taken to elicit all the factors that might be contributing to a child's disorder before an accurate diagnosis and formulation is made and an intervention planned.

Psychological symptoms in children are common, as shown by epidemiological studies. They present to GPs, paediatricians and community medical officers with only one-tenth of children who suffer from a psychiatric disorder finding their way to a child psychiatrist. Psychiatric disorder in children can be defined as an abnormality of behaviour, emotion or relationships sufficiently marked and prolonged to cause handicap to the child himself or herself, and/or distress and disturbance in the family and community. Rutter's important study (1988) used questionnaires to measure the prevalence of psychiatric disorder among 10–11-year olds living on the Isle of Wight. He found an overall rate of 6.8% which was broken down further to give a prevalence of 4.0% for conduct disorder and a prevalence of 2.5% for emotional disorder.

Other findings can be summarized as follows:

1 Sex ratio—twofold excess of boys.
2 An association between reading retardations and conduct disorder.
3 An increase in prevalence in children with chronic physical disorders.
4 A substantial increase if a brain disorder is present. This in certain age ranges could be as much as a fivefold increase.
5 Increased prevalence in those children who have learning difficulties.

At the younger end of the age range Richman et al. (1978) found a prevalence of 7% of moderate and marked disorders in a sample of 3-year olds. In adolescence, it is generally agreed that the prevalence is between 10–15% although it has been found to be higher in some studies.

Developmental aspects of psychiatric disorder in childhood and adolescence

Children are developing human beings and because of this a thorough knowledge of child development is essential when working in any field involving children. This is especially true when considering psychiatric disorder in children, as the age of the child will determine the presenting symptoms which are dependent on both the emotional and cognitive developmental stage of the child.

Psychological symptoms may not be of concern at one age, but might cause concern if they are either persistent or are seen occuring at an inappropriate developmental age. There are many examples of this. For instance, sleep problems are very common in pre-school children and would not be considered a sign of disorder at that age, but in an older child they would be, and therefore are likely to be more significant. In the same way, an 8-year old might be diagnosed as enuretic, but bedwetting in a 3-year old would not be of significance and would be entirely expected in a 2-year old. For the common psychological symptoms presenting at different ages see Table 3. Note, these are common problems and not disorders as defined above.

Classification

The diagnostic categories of psychiatric disorder in childhood and adolescence are defined descriptively. It is rare to make a diagnosis of formal mental illness under the age of 16, but nevertheless the daignosis and treatment of such illness is an important part of the work of the child psychiatrist. The clinical syndromes specific to childhood and adolescence have been described in the World Health Organisation's International Classification of Disease 9 (ICD9). In order to take account of all the factors operating in psychological disturbance in childhood a multi-axial classification has been devised. This uses five different axes:

1 clinical psychiatric syndrome;
2 specific delays in development;

Table 3 Common psychological symptoms in childhood—a different symptomatology according to age

Age	Types of behaviour complained of	Other problems

0–5	Tantrums
	Oppositional and
	  negative behaviour
	Aggression
		Feeding
		Sleeping
		Developmental delay
		Separation anxiety
		  (clinginess)

5–11	Lying Stealing Fighting Disobedience	Fears Phobias Nightmares Soiling Problems with peers
11–16	Fighting Stealing Truancy Running away Disobedience Substance abuse	School refusal Anxiety and depression Moodiness Social withdrawal Difficulties with peers

3   intellectual level;
4   physical problems; and
5   abnormal social situations.

Disorders in pre-school children

There is no classification of pre-school disorders yet defined and the usual presentation at this age is with difficult behaviour. The behaviour complained of is most often home based as children of this age are still very dependent on their parents, but the behaviour may also be observed in other situations, such as the nursery, e.g. aggressive behaviour with peers. The sorts of behaviours complained of are sleep problems, negative and oppositional behaviour, feeding difficulties and, as already mentioned, aggressive behaviour. At this age behaviour patterns are not well established and intervention can be very successful by improving the parents' management of the child and the parent–child relationship. Constitutional factors such as developmental delay, autism (this is rare) and other neurobiological disorders should be identified and assessed so that appropriate treatment or educational provision can be made. The psychiatrist also needs to be able to comment on the attachment of children to their adult carers and this can be done by observing attachment behaviour. Before the age of 6 months a baby is not likely to protest if held by a stranger, but after that age anxiety with stranger is the norm and the baby will protest if separated from his or her mother. When mobile he or she will use the mother as a base from which to explore. Abnormal attachment behaviour can be either lack of anxiety when presented with a stranger and inappropriate displays of affection or clingy behaviour which suggest an anxious attachement. After the age of 3 years attachment behaviour is less easy to observe but problems may persist due to poor attachment in early childhood.

Autism is a clinical syndrome which presents in early childhood and is recognized by abnormalities of speech and language as well as severe impairment in the child's ability to make social relationships. It also includes compulsive and ritualistic behaviours. Modern theories of aetiology suggest a biological basis to the syndrome. Disintegrative psychosis is not seen as early as autism and is always associated with an organic brain disorder.

Common psychiatric syndromes presenting in childhood

Conduct disorders

There are a number of definitions of conduct disorder but they all make reference to the antisocial nature of the disorder. The disorder is characterized by such behaviour as stealing, persistent lying, truancy, running away, aggression and disobedience. In girls aggression may be less of a problem but staying out, overdosing and promiscuity are common.

The factors implicated in the aetiology of the disorder are multiple and can be divided simply into: those within the family, those within the child and those found in the wider environment and community. Factors operating in the family are: poor early attachments, inconsistent handling with poor control, marital discord and one-parent families. Factors in the child include difficult temperamental styles and the presence of physical disorder such as brain damage, developmental delay or epilepsy. Within the environment the cultural influences on parenting, the school attended and social disadvantage can all influence the level of antisocial behaviour in a community.

The prognosis varies but is poor in children with severe, persistent symptoms, and these children can be difficult to treat. They tend to make poor relationships as adults and continue to show antisocial and criminal behaviour. They also have a high incidence of psychiatric illness in adulthood.

Emotional disorders

Emotional disorders in childhood are characterized by symptoms of anxiety, fearfulness, misery and unhappiness. They bear some resemblance to adult neuroses but the syndromes are not well differentiated. The prognosis is good with little persistence of symptoms into adult life. A common symptom seen in these children is anxiety, and a common cause of anxiety in middle childhood is fear of losing a parent. This can be looked at in terms of family dynamics and a likely pattern of interaction would be as separation anxiety on the part of the child and overinvolvement on the part of the parent. Treatment is often aimed at creating an appropriate distance between parent and child. Separation anxiety is more important component of school refusal than school-based problems. However, having said that, these children may find it hard to cope with the demands of school both academically and because of difficulty in coping with peer relationships.

Depression in childhood may be difficult to diagnose, and questionnaires have been developed which can detect its presence. If biological symptoms are present then small doses of antidepressants may be helpful. In most cases, however, treatment which aims to help resolve the causes of the child's misery and unhappiness is successful and in practice medication is rarely used. Sometimes treatment will need to help the child come to terms with painful issues such as school bullying or the separation of his or her parents and this may involve individual therapy or may need the involvement of the family in family therapy. This is often the approach when grief is an issue for a family.

Child abuse (see below) usually produces marked emotional disorder.

Developmental disorders

Elimination disorders

Enuresis

Primary nocturnal enuresis is very common and is a developmental disorder resulting from the slow maturation of the nervous system. There is often a family history of this complaint. The most successful treatment is the enuresis alarm. There can be secondary psychological disturbance if the child is viewed negatively by his parents and they are excessively punitive. Bedwetting in itself will not normally require intervention by a psychiatrist.

Encopresis

Persistent faecal soiling after the age of 4 years may well need the involvement of psychiatric help. It can be divided into retentive or non-retentive and it is usual to find it occurring in the context of a disturbed relationship between parent and child, if poor toilet training has been excluded as a cause. A careful history will distinguish the two. Poor training is usually associated with general inadequate parenting, whereas a disturbed parent–child relationship will be revealed by the parent's description of the child's behaviour. The soiling can be seen as an aggressive act directed at the parents. Treatment will depend on the type of soiling, how entrenched it has become and the factors responsible for its cause. The sorts of interventions that can be brought to bear are behavioural techniques that will involve the use of rewards for appropriate use of the toilet, family therapy which aims at changing family patterns of interaction and which looks at the purpose that the symptom is serving for the family and, if the symptom is entrenched, then individual psychotherapy may be necessary. In-patient treatment is occasionally needed when out-patient strategies fail. Prognosis will vary according to the type of soiling and its severity but in the majority of cases it does not persist beyond the mid-teens.

Other developmental disorders

Other developmental disorders which may be seen in child psychiatric practice include specific learning disorders, speech and language disorders and hyper-activity.

Overactivity is a commonly-seen symptom in children and may be due to a number of causes such as anxiety, poor control by parents and frustration. The true hyperkinetic syndrome with pervasive overactivity, distractability and impulsivity is rare. The Americans recognize a syndrome, attention deficit disorder, which consists of distractability, short attention span and impulsivity with or without motor hyperactivity. It is important to look carefully at the behaviour the parent is complaining about as parents will often label a child hyperactive when the child is disobedient, disruptive and lacking in controls.

Adolescence

Adolescence is a time of transition when an individual moves from childhood to adulthood and it is therefore a major developmental stage which results not only in emotional upheaval for the individual but also represents an important time in the life cycle of the family who have to negotiate the departure (emotionally if not physically) of one of their members. The adolescent also has to cope with the physical changes of puberty and these themselves can be a considerable source of stress. Epidemiological studies which have asked adolescents to report their feelings have confirmed that for many, adolescence is a time of emotional turmoil.

Disorders presenting in adolescence can be simply divided into unresolved childhood disorders, incipient adult-type disorders and those disorders related to the stresses of puberty and adolescence itself. Some general observations regarding disturbance related to the stresses of puberty and adolescence follow: It should be noted that anorexia nervosa is a condition which is seen mainly in adolescents and this is described on p. 94. There has been much discussion about how much rebelliousness is normal in adolescents, and while some young people and their families seem to negotiate this difficult time with apparent ease, other young people seem to need to test their family's endurance to the limit. It would appear that a family's ability to be supportive, tolerant and flexible and yet provide the right amount of security and control will determine how successful they are in launching their young people into the world. The behaviour with which adolescents present can be very disturbing to those around them, not only to their family but also to teachers and other professionals involved with their care. It can also be a source of anxiety and distress for the young people themselves. These disturbing behaviours can include truancy, academic failure, running away, substance abuse, promiscuity and suicide attempts. Other young people report feelings of unhappiness and misery and will tend to withdraw from their family and friends.

Those involved with such disturbing young people (social worker or psychiatrist) will need to be flexible: most of these problems need a 'whole family approach' (i.e. an analysis of the family dynamics), as it is in the context of family life that the difficulties are arising. In some cases, however, the adolescent will need space outside the family to try to resolve his or her difficulties and then individual therapy may be appropriate, or even inpatient treatment if the problems are sufficiently severe. Suicidal behaviour in adolescents should always be taken seriously and can produce a useful crisis from which real change can result within a family. A family interview should always be part of the assessment of an adolescent who has attempted suicide.

Psychoses

Childhood schizophrenia is extremely rare and has a similar symptomatology to the adult schizophrenias. Schizophrenia is rather more common after puberty when it is more likely to resemble the adult illness. Accurate diagnosis is important because of the *consequences of diagnosis*. In these types of disorders medication is a major part of treatment but also the role of the family in providing support and security should not be forgotten. Indeed, certain family behaviours are as potent at preventing schizophrenic relapse as phenothiazines are.

Child abuse

Under this heading are included the physical abuse of children by beating, battering, burning and other similar gross assaults. Sexual abuse is also included and in general the same principles apply.

The 'battered child syndrome' was first described in 1868 by a professor of legal medicine in Paris, but it was not until the 1960s that doctors came to accept that the many injuries that they had attributed to pathology, such as rickets, were in fact due to often repeated injury by an adult, usually the parent(s).

Similarly, with sexual abuse, there is now a greater awareness of the nature and extent of the problem, but resistance to acknowledging its magnitude is still considerable.

People continue to harbour certain misconceptions about abuse. They think it is only the poor who abuse, but this is not so. Abuse crosses class boundaries. They think abusive parents are all incurably abnormal, psychotic, criminal or retarded. This is only true of a small percentage of them. The majority are rather unhappy people who feel desperately guilty about their failure to behave as loving parents and who crave for and respond to support. The third misconception is that it is a rare phenomenon. In the USA in 1978 child abuse of all kinds was being reported 320 times per million of the population, but it is now known that this was just a fraction of the total. A similar picture emerges in Britain with cases being identified at an earlier, more 'treatable' stage. The abused generally grow up to abuse unless appropriate intervention can be offered. Ruth and Henry Kempe in their study of child abuse came to the conclusion that four out of five abusers could be helped and that only 10%, which included the mentally ill, sociopaths and those with mental handicap were untreatable (Kempe & Kempe, 1978).

They devised a method of predicting child abusers from the earliest stage, when the parents' attitudes to the immediate birth of their child plus their immediate response to the birth could be noted. They also drew up a checklist of things in a parent's background which would suggest a greater potential for abuse. They saw this approach as providing support at the most appropriate time. Treatment included a mixture of therapy, crisis intervention and support through lay volunteers. In all forms of child abuse, close coordination between child psychiatrists and social workers (who are mainly involved) is essential.

Sexual abuse can range from indecent exposure to full intercourse. The fact that there is no physical evidence of abuse does not mean that it has not taken place nor that it will be of less significance to the victim. The longer the abuse is allowed to continue the greater the psychological damage.

Abusers are generally known by their victims. Children very rarely lie about the fact that they have been abused and their account should be treated seriously. The fact that a child later retracts her/his allegation does not mean the abuse never happened. A sensitive multi-disciplinary approach and well thought-out procedure can often avoid such denial occurring. There is a higher percentage of female than male victims, thought the picture is changing as more boys are starting to talk about being abused. Children who have been abused either show physical signs, e.g. vaginal scarring, bruising, irritation or chronic urinary tract infection, or their behaviour changes in some way. They become clingy, tearful, secretive, unhappy about uncovering their bodies and moody. They may show a premature awareness of things sexual and their play may revolve around sexual activities. Some abused children become sexually provocative themselves and thus expose themselves to further risk of abuse. Practitioners should not fall into the common trap of accepting the argument, used in mitigation by abusers, that the victim encouraged and enjoyed the abuse. Therapists should keep in mind that the adult abuser has betrayed his position of trust and authority in relation to a minor and taken advantage either of the child's inferior physical strength or of the child's trust in that adult.

Rehabilitation of the abuser back into the family home, if it was the father for example, is not successful unless the abuser can admit his guilt, and this may be just the start of a reorganization of the 'balance of power' within the family. Generally a strengthening of the bond between child and mother has to be created before rehabilitation can take place. So far, treatment of sexual abusers has met with only limited success. Diagnosis and assessment of child abuse is often very difficult, but inaction through fear of making a mistake or breaking up the family can, in the long run, cause greater unhappiness. 'Failure to treat the victims has far more serious social consequences than failure to punish the perpetrator.' (Kempe & Kempe 1978).

References

Kempe, R. S. & Kempe, C. H. (1978) *Child Abuse*. Fortuna, London.

Richman, N., Stevenson, J. & Graham, P. (1978) Prevalence of behaviour problems in 3 year old children: an epidemiological study in a London borough. *Journal of Child Psychology and Psychiatry*, **16**, 222–87.

Rutter, M. (1988) *Developmental Psychiatry*. Cambridge University Press, Cambridge.

Further reading

Bentovim, A. *et al.* (1988) *Child Sexual Abuse: Assessment and Treatment*. John Wright, Bristol.

Erikson, E. (1967) *Childhood and Society*. Pelican, London.

Rutter, M. (1977) *Helping Troubled Children*. Pelican, London.

Winnicott, D. W. (1970) *The Child, the Family and the Outside World*. Pelican, London.

Wolff, S. (1971) *Children Under Stress*. Penguin, London.

Chapter 10
Eating Disorders

Introduction

Eating disorders include anorexia nervosa and bulimia. The earliest description of anorexia nervosa was in 1649 by Richard Morton who called it 'nervous consumption'. It was later described in more detail by Sir William Gull in the late nineteenth century. These disorders are becoming more common. Some investigators report that that between 5% and 10% of adolescent girls develop one or other variety of eating disorder.

Between the 1950s and 1970s in Switzerland the incidence of anorexia nervosa went up from 0.38 to 1.12 per 100 000. In this country Crisp *et al.* (1976) have put the prevalence rate of anorexia nervosa in English private schools at around 1%. Approximately 90% of anorexic and bulimic patients are female and tend to come from middle class families.

Clinical features

It is customary to discuss anorexia and bulimia separately but it should be realized that the conditions may coexist. Some bulimic patients give a clear history of anorexia nervosa and others drift from bulimia into permanent anorexia.

Anorexia nervosa usually starts in a teenage girl who is afraid that she is overweight. This leads to slimming, purging and food refusal. Curiously enough although the word anorexia is used, most anorexic patients have a perfectly normal appetite, it is just that they are terrified of eating.

Undoubtedly cultural influences are of great importance with the current emphasis on slimming which can quite easily become pathological. It is likely that the majority of young women become excessively preoccupied with weight control and that if they are vulnerable or immature then they will become anorexic.

The criteria by which anorexia nervosa is diagnosed include the following features:

1 A refusal to maintain minimal body weight; weight loss leading to maintenance of body weight 15% below the expected weight.

2 Intense fear of becoming or appearing obese even when obviously underweight.

3 Disturbance in the way in which the person perceives the body image. This can easily be demonstrated using a simple analogue scale.

4 In female patients, amenorrhoea for at least 3 months.

Anorexia nervosa is a life-threatening illness; the usual mortality rate is quoted as being between 5% and 10% but higher mortality rates have been reported from Sweden. Patients may develop dangerously low potassium levels and require intravenous fluid therapy upon admission to hospital, although conditions of this severity are not especially common. The complications that result from anorexia nervosa are simply those of plain starvation including such features as anaemia, low blood pressure, cardiac arrhythmias, renal stones and osteoporosis. The differential diagnosis of the condition includes the exclusion of disorders such as tuberculosis, malignant disease and hypopituitarism. Psychiatric disorders which may mimic anorexia include schizophrenia, depression and obsessional states.

Bulimic disorder tends to come on later than anorexia and is characterized by:

1   Recurrent episodes of binge eating where the person consumes huge quantities of food in a relatively short period of time.

2   Fear of being unable to stop eating during the binges.

3   Self-induced vomiting, laxative and diuretic use or rigorous exercise, etc. to avoid weight gain.

4   A minimum average of two binge eating episodes per week for 3 months.

5   Persistent over-preoccupation with body shape and weight.

A useful physical sign is abrasion of the knuckles caused by self-induced vomiting (Russell's sign).

Treatment

The treatment of anorexia nervosa is difficult. In the past many favoured a psychotherapeutic approach, but overviews of treatment indicate that probably the most successful treatment is acceptance of the fact that the person will relapse and need frequent readmission to hospital with the development of good therapeutic relationships with the nursing staff and supervised feeding. Behavioural techniques have been used in which the patient is admitted to a room which is stripped of everything except for a bed and minimal furniture. The patient has no privileges, but a hierarchical list of privileges is drawn up and the patient earns a privilege, e.g. being allowed to clean her teeth, by consuming a meal and then gradually works through to the stage where she is able to receive visitors, go out, etc. It seems surprising that people tolerate this regime, but they do. Pharmacotherapy has a place in the management of anorexia and in this instance some favour the use of chlorpromazine, others the use of tricyclic antidepressants. Dosage may have to be low at first because of the person's extremely low weight.

It is rarely necessary to resort to tube feeding but with a narrow gauge nasogastric tube it is possible to give a person 3000 calories a day with minimal discomfort as opposed to the horrors of old-fashioned tube feeding.

Bulimic patients tend to be older and come to treatment much later than anorexic patients. Again a variety of treatment methods have been used including individual and group therapy. In the group, emphasis is placed on re-education in eating habits more than anything else.

In all eating disorders the family will need to be brought in to the treatment process even though full-scale family therapy may not be needed. Very often the family will deny that the patient has had such a disorder and in the case of anorexics the patient is often the source of family admiration for her ability to 'control herself'. Interestingly enough, when anorexic patients improve it is common to find that one or other parent may develop a significant degree of depression.

Whatever methods are used, the psychiatrist must recognize the tendency towards relapse and chronicity and be prepared for repeated readmission. In general, outpatient treatment in severe cases is not indicated. In the author's experience the key to successful treatment lies very much in the hands of the nursing staff who, by working in specialized units, will have developed the patience and forbearance to deal with an extremely difficult group of patients to contain within a therapeutic relationship.

A prospective study of the appearance of ballet dancers, athletes and models through the years could aid our understanding of anorexia.

Reference

Crisp, A. H., Palmer, R. L. & Kalucy, R. S. (1976) How common is anorexia nervosa?: a prevalence study. *British Journal of Psychiatry*, **128**, 549–54.

Further reading

Garfinkel, P. E. & Garner, D. M. (1982) *Anorexia Nervosa: a Multidimensional Perspective*. Brunner-Mazel, New York.

Russell, G. F. M. (1977) Editorial: the present status of anorexia nervosa. *Psychological Medicine*, **7**, 363–7.

Russell, G. F. M. (1979) Bulimia nervosa: an ominous variant of anorexia nervosa. *Psychological Medicine*, **9**, 429.

Chapter 11
Psychiatric Disorders in the Elderly

Introduction

If youth and adolescence are times of emotional development, maturation and turbulence, so old age is, psychologically speaking, a time of relative stability. However, this relative stability is often more apparent than real and it should be realized that old age often brings psychological difficulties. Quite apart from this the elderly face special physical and social problems.

Once people become old the physical aspects and hazards of ageing become apparent. Their joints and skin lose their elasticity and they become prone to those common disorders of the heart and circulation which are such an important feature of the morbidity of the 60–70 age group. It is unfortunate that at this time of life the average person usually undergoes a major social change, e.g. retirement or widowhood. There are, therefore, obvious sources of stress in old age which merit enumeration:

1 Deteriorating physical health, e.g. hypertension, ichaemic heart disease, chronic bronchitis.
2 Poverty.
3 Loneliness.
4 Loss of a marital partner.
5 Altered social role in a competitive society.
6 Fear of death.
7 Malnutrition.

The particular psychological disadvantage of the old person is a lack of flexibility.

In old age personality traits are already well established and patterns of behaviour relatively fixed. It is a commonplace finding that rigidity of outlook and feeling are part of the normal manifestations of ageing.

It is, therefore, always important to bear this in mind when trying to assess the mental state of a supposedly abnormal elderly patient. A certain stubborness and obstinacy which may be normal in the elderly person may be given undue value by a prejudiced or inexperienced observer.

It is a common fallacy that there is a loss of intellectual ability with age. Current measures of intelligence stress new learning at the expense of experience which is very difficult to measure as well as being very varied in its nature. Psychometry thus puts a premium on 'cross-sectional' or 'latitudinal' intelligence and discounts experiental or 'longitudinal' intelligence. In fact this latter shows insignificant decline with healthy ageing. This is in contrast to new learning, a relatively unimportant part of intellect in the educated, experienced person.

Psychiatric syndromes

From what has been stated above it will be clear that the special features of psychiatric syndromes in the elderly are related to the fact that the individual's personality is fixed, his or her capacity for change limited and hence, often, his or her reaction to a situation more calamitous than if he or she were 20 years younger.

Affective disorders

These are the most important group of illnesses to consider because these depressive states (involutional melancholia) are so amenable to treatment. It is therefore doubly important that the depressed elderly patient is not overlooked. It is easy to mistake a state of chronic apathetic depression and suppose that an individual is a lonely old person when in fact he or she is a lonely, depressed old person. At all events the syndrome is notable for:

1   profound depressive affect;
2   striking degrees of agitation; and
3   massive ideas of guilt and self-recrimination, often of delusional intensity.

This variety of affective disorder is not difficult to diagnose. However, lesser degrees of depression may be. One should, therefore, always be on the lookout for the apathy, hypochondriasis, inertia and sleep disturbance associated with depression.

Hypomanic excitement

In the elderly this is not uncommon but is apt to be persistent and again may go unrecognized if not severe, e.g. an 86-year-old man was said to be presenting a difficult problem in management in a geriatric ward because of his interfering, restless behaviour. He was described as 'thieving and mischievous'. In fact, on examination he presented a typical picture of mild hypomanic excitement with elation and some grandiose ideas. All this settled with appropriate medication.

Treatment

Antidepressant medication is the treatment of choice though severely depressed old people will respond very well to ECT providing their physical conditions permit it.

Imipramine and amitriptyline are the most frequently used anti-depressants in the elderly. Caution should be exercised in commencing these medications since the usual initial dose of 25 mg tds may induce states of excitement, or in the case of amitriptyline, excessive drowsiness. It is therefore advisable to start off with 10 mg tds.

Paranoid psychoses

Acute paranoid reactions are commonly encountered in the elderly. The patient may develop an acute illness in which agitation and presecutory notions are prominent. In many instances a strong *affective colouring* is found, whilst in others there may be evidence of *organic impairment*. Sensory deficits such as impaired hearing may also contribute to the problem. Whatever the aetiology it is important to recognize that these acute disturbances, if handled carefully and sensibly, will have a favourable outcome.

The reaction may have been triggered off by some obvious event in the patient's life, such as removal from home to an old people's home, or admission to hospital. Such a change of environment may be too much for the old person who then becomes frightened, suspicious and bewildered, and if treated tactlessly, even by well-meaning individuals, may 'blow up' into a state of psychotic excitement.

Aetiology

Many paranoid syndromes in the elderly arise as an acute reaction set against a background of organic cerebral impairment. This is most commonly associated with either *cerebral arteriosclerosis* or *senile dementia*. Others are heavily coloured by affective symptoms and are probably *affective in origin*. They respond well to anti-depressive treatment.

It should be remembered too that the old person *handicapped by deafness or blindness* is a likely candidate for a paranoid state.

Schizophrenic psychoses can arise in the elderly — these are little different in form from other schizophrenias. Finally the paranoid syndrome may be grafted on to a *lifelong paranoid personality disorder*.

Organic syndromes

Organic syndromes including subacute delirious states superimposed on dementia are commonplace in the elderly. It is not uncommon for such patients to require admission to hospital in an acutely disturbed state in which disorientation and restlessness are manifest.

Aetiology

A typical clinical picture is one of acute confusion with perplexity, restlessness, incoherence of thought and feeling. The most common setting for this is either *cerebral arteriosclerosis* or *Alzheimer's dementia*, but in addition to this *acute confusional episodes in the elderly* can be caused by such events as myocardial infarction, bronchopneumonia, anaemia and uraemia. These four conditions should always be borne in mind. They are easily excluded and investigations aimed at this should be routine in the examination of the confused elderly person.

General considerations

Any elderly person who develops a psychiatric syndrome should be carefully evaluated in his or her home situation before the decision is taken to admit to a psychiatric hospital. Admission to hospital should only be arranged if there is a clear indication, i.e. if the patient can best be treated in hospital. It is vital that the elderly patient should not lose his or her place in the community. Whitehead has demonstrated convincingly the value of psychiatric admissions on a 'month in and month out' basis even with quite severely demented patients. In addition to this the elderly patient with psychiatric disturbance can be perfectly adequately maintained at day hospitals, or day centres.

The patient's physical health should be carefully investigated and disorders such as chronic bronchitis, ischaemic heart disease, prostatic enlargement and arthritis all searched for and given adequate treatment.

Of course, there are some patients who will require long-term care in hospital, e.g. those with severe states of dementia, but these should be in the minority. Local authorities provide residential accommodation for patients with psychogeriatric disturbance and these services should be utilized wherever possible.

Although in many instances the goals of psychiatric treatment in the elderly patient may be limited, the results are, nonetheless, often extremely gratifying. The dramatic relief of the previously unrecognized depression can cause a radical alteration in the patient's way of life. Simple psychotherapy, too, is of great value. It is easy to avoid old people and all too often they are ignored and retreat into mild, hostile apathy. Simple discussion of their problems, acknowledgement of their status and awareness of their plight with sympathetic understanding can always produce considerable symptomatic relief.

Further reading

Corsellis, J. A. N. (1962) *Mental Illness and the Ageing Brain*. Maudsley Monograph 9. Oxford University Press, Oxford.

Guardian, the (1985) Old Soldiers Never Die. 3/1/85, 14/3/85, 25/10/85.

Post, F. (1962) *The Significance of Affective Symptoms in old Age*. Maudsley Monography 10. Oxford University Press, Oxford.

Praag, H. van (1977) Psychotropic drugs in the aged. *Comprehensive Psychiatry*, **18**, 429.

Chapter 12
Psychiatry and the Law: The Mental Health Act, 1983

Historical background

The history of the care of the mentally ill is on the whole a grim story consisting mainly of neglect, indifference and ill treatment, despite islands of progress. From time to time reforming persons halted this process, and laws were passed to regulate the running of asylums for the insane and protect inmates.

The main purpose of such institutions was custodial—if a patient entered, he or she stood only a small chance of returning to the world since little active treatment could be offered and society did not welcome his or her return, believing the patient to be dangerous and beyond hope of improvement.

The nineteenth century saw emphasis on the moral treatment of the insane, i.e. treating patients like human beings, and a great deal was accomplished to improve the care of patients, finding them useful occupations, removing restraint and encouraging a more hopeful attitude.

Nevertheless legislation was cumbersome, and even as late as 1890 the passage of the Lunacy Acts did not make the position easier. If anything the mental hospitals were fixed in a custodial role, since voluntary admission to mental hospital was impossible. A step forward occurred in 1930, with the Mental Treatment Act, which enabled people to enter hospital voluntarily. In the past 20 years, as knowledge and therapeutic zeal increased, it became apparent that a less unwieldy set of laws was needed. This culminated in the 1959 Mental Health Act which represented a high-point of humane and caring practice, transferring mental health firmly from the legal to the medical arena. However, it was felt, especially by patients' organizations, that paternalistic power in the hands of psychiatrists was worse than legal process. A compromise, the 1983 Mental Health Act, brought in the Mental Health Act Commission, second opinions and a variety of measures designed to protect the liberties of the patient.

Currently further refinement, to permit compulsory treatment to be given in the community, is being debated.

The Mental Health Act, 1983

This is a comprehensive act slightly modifying the 1959 Act and repealing the Lunacy Acts of 1890 and the Mental Treatment Act of 1930. The most important general features of the 1959 and 1983 Acts are as follows:

1   Control of mental hospitals and mental nursing homes, etc. passes from the Board of Control to the National Health Service. (Introduced 1959.)

2   Informal admission of patients is encouraged. (Introduced 1959.)

3   The procedure surrounding compulsory admission to hospital is made more clinical and less formal and intimidating. (Introduced 1959.)

4 The role of the local authority in mental health services is defined. (Introduced 1959.)

5 A Mental Health Act Commission that can inspect hospitals, hear patients' complaints and appoint second opinions to cases is brought in. (Introduced 1983.)

The Act is divided into ten parts:

Part 1 states the application of the Act and defines mental disorder. It includes mental illness, mental impairment (previously known as mental handicap) and psychopathic disorder. Sexual deviation, immorality and addiction to alcohol or other drugs are excluded as reasons for applying the Act. (s. 1)

Part 2 deals with compulsory admission to hospital and guardianship. (s. 2–34)

Part 3 deals with patients concerned in criminal proceedings or under sentence. (s. 35–55)

Part 4 deals with consent to treatment. Certain treatments, deemed hazardous (e.g. ECT), require consent of the patient *or* an independent second opinion agreeing with the first. Other treatments, deemed irreversible (e.g. psycho-surgery) require consent *and* an agreeing second opinion. (s. 56–64)

Part 5 deals with Mental Health Review Tribunals. A patient can appeal against his or her detention and be heard or legally represented at such a tribunal. The responsible medical officer (RMO) may be required to give evidence to the tribunal and the tribunal may direct the patient's discharge. (s. 65–79)

Part 6 concerns the removal and return of patients within differing legal jurisdictions (e.g. England, Scotland and Ireland). (s. 80–92)

Part 7 outlines the management of the property and affairs of patients. (s. 93–113)

Part 8 empowers specially trained and approved social workers, lays down the provision of a code of practice and creates the Mental Health Act Commission. (s. 114–125)

Part 9 deals with offences against the Act. (s. 126–130)

Part 10 contains miscellaneous provisions. (s. 131–149)

The sections of the Act of most interest to medical students are the first five.

Section 2

Section 2 is used to detain a patient for a period not exceeding 28 days for purposes of observation and treatment. The patient has the right of appeal to a tribunal within 14 days of admission.

Section 3

Section 3 is used to detain a patient for treatment for up to 6 months. It can be overruled by the patient's next of kin.

In sections 2 and 3 two medical recommendations are needed. One should be the patient's own general practitioner and the other should be a doctor, specially qualified under section 12 of the Act. The medical officers must examine the patient and satisfy themselves that he or she presents a danger to him or herself or others by reason of mental disorder. In addition, if the grounds for detention are psychopathic disorder or mental impairment, the responsible medical officer must consider the patient treatable.

Section 4

Section 4 provides for the emergency admission of a patient by one medical recommendation for a period of 72 hours pending further action. Sections 2, 3 and 4 then require an application by a next of kin or social worker, which medical recommendation supports.

Section 5

Section 5 empowers the emergency detention by the RMO of an already admitted patient for a further 72 hours. The nurse in charge of the patient may apply a holding order, until the medical officer is available, for a maximum of 6 hours.

Criminal responsibility

It is an established principle of English law that a man or woman is responsible for his or her own actions — that is to say that he/she intends their result. Therefore it follows that in the eyes of the law he/she must bear the responsibility for them. In the case of serious offences, responsibility is the more likely to be questioned. In the case of an individual suffering from mental illness committing a crime, it has been argued for many years that the person's state of mind must impair responsibility for his or her acts. This has, however, not been easy to establish in a court of law since the law assumes everyone is sane, and insanity has to be poven. Since 1843 the courts have used the MacNaughten Rules as a test of insanity. These rules arose following the trial for murder of Daniel MacNaughten who killed Sir Robert Peel's private secretary. MacNaughten had paranoid delusions and was acquitted on the direction of the judge.

Subsequently judges formulated the rules as they have been known ever since, as a series of answers to questions put to them by the House of Lords. In practice the rules seek the answers to the questions:

1   Regarding the offence, did the accused know the nature and quality of the act?

2   If he did, did he know he was doing wrong?

Clearly if the patient were deluded the answer to **1** may be 'yes' but to **2** 'no'.

Despite their apparent simplicity, the rules can be difficult to apply and make for only a limited acknowledgement of impaired responsibility. For years they have been the subject of controversy, both here and in the USA. Nevertheless they are still widely applied as tests of insanity in capital cases.

Since the Homicide Act of 1959 the law in England and Wales has acknowledged the concept of diminished responsibility, which can be invoked if an accused person is shown to be suffering from 'such abnormality of mind . . . as substantially to impair his responsibility'. The concept of diminished responsibility has not been accepted without reserve, and it has been pointed out that once allowance is made for diminished responsibility one is calling into question the whole idea of criminal responsibility at any level.

Testamentary capacity

The ability to make a valid will depends on the possession of 'sound disposing mind'. This is not defined in law but the concept is derived from the notion that the person concerned should fulfill the following criteria: he or she should understand the implications of the act of making a will, have a good idea of the extent of the estate and know who are the likely beneficiaries. Mental illness, whether through psychosis or organic cerebral disease, does not automatically debar someone from making a valid will, since even in chronic schizophrenia and in dementia there are often well-preserved areas of lucidity and contact with reality. A doctor should never witness a will irrespective of whether or not he or she is a beneficiary.

Fitness to plead

A defendant is fit to plead if he or she:
1   knows the difference between right and wrong;
2   understands the difference between a plea of guilty and one of 'innocent';
3   can instruct a lawyer in his or her defence; and
4   can challenge a juror.

If unfit the defendant has an automatic defence of not guilty by reason of insanity, but the penalty, fixed by law, of detention at Her Majesty's pleasure (section 41) is so severe that it is not an intelligent defence when lesser penalties are available under different sections of the Act. Usually therefore *actus reus* is established and the court seeks a medical opinion and recommendation.

Court reports

A medical officer is often called upon to provide expert witness orally, or in writing, upon a case. In writing, the report should begin by stating the basis of the report, e.g. 'This report is based upon one examination of the defendant at Newtown Police Station and my reading of his case records at Oldtown Hospital. I have not seen any depositions.' 'Depositions' is the name given to the written statements deposited as evidence by the prosecution and defence lawyers before the court. It is reasonable always to ask for the prosecution depositions before writing a report and also for the defence depositions if they are requesting the report.

The report should then describe succinctly the *alleged* material events. The events should be referred to as alleged, for the court will not accept hearsay. After a further brief biographical paragraph on the patient, the report should conclude with an opinion. This should state clearly:
1   whether the patient is under disability at law (fit to plead);
2   whether he or she is suffering from a mental disorder within the meaning of the Mental Health Act 1983;

Table 4 Summary of the names of orders directing detention with corresponding section number of the 1983 Mental Health Act

Duration	Section number	Order	Applicants
28 days	2	Assessment order (civil)	2 doctors + NOK or SW
6 months + 6 months + 12 months + ...	3	Treatment order (civil)	2 doctors + NOK or SW
72 hours	4	Emergency order	1 doctor + NOK or SW
6 hours	5	Holding order	C/N (RMO)
3 × 28 days	35	Assessment remand	1 doctor + judge
3 × 28 days	36	Treatment remand	2 doctors + judge
6 months + 6 months + 12 months + ...	37	Treatment order (judicial)	2 doctors + judge
12 weeks + N (28 days) < 6 months	38	Assessment order (judicial)	2 doctors + judge
Indefinite	41	Restriction order	2 doctors + judge
RMO and independent doctor + PSW + C/N	57	Irreversible treatment certificate	Consent and 2nd opinion
RMO and independent doctor + PSW + C/N	58	Hazardous treatment certificate	Consent or 2nd opinion
72 hours	136	Police order	Police constable

C/N = charge nurse; NOK = next of kin; PSW = psychiatric social worker; RMO = responsible medical officer; SW = social worker.

3 whether, if he or she is not mentally disordered, another condition exists, e.g. alcohol addiction, that is amenable to medical intervention; and
4 whether there is any medical recommendation for the court to consider (e.g. assessment remand section 35, treatment order section 37).

One should state whether or not one is specially approved under the Act for the purpose of such reports and sign with one's full qualifications and status.

Some names of detention orders are given in Table 4.

Further reading

Butler Report (1975) *Mentally Abnormal Offenders.* Her Majesty's Stationery office, Cmnd 6244.

Gibbens, T. C. N. (1974) Preparing psychiatric court reports. *British Journal of Hospital Medicine,* 278–84.

Mack, J. E. (1975) *Borderline States in Psychiatry.* Grune & Stratton, New York.

Walker, N. (1965) *Crime and Punishment.* Churchill Livingstone, Edinburgh.

West, D. J. (1982) Delinquency: its roots, careers and prospects. In L. Radzinowicz (Ed.) *Cambridge Studies in Criminology.* Heinemann, London.

Up to date reviews of psychiatry and the laws are to be found in the regular articles on forensic psychiatry in the *British Journal of Hospital Medicine,* e.g. Fenwick, P. B. C. (1986) Automatism and the law. *British Journal of Hospital Medicine,* **36,** 397.

Chapter 13
Treatment in Psychiatry

Introduction

The term 'treatment' is used in a wide sense in psychiatry; specific remedies for illnesses of known aetiology are practically unknown, so treatment tends to be empirical and eclectic. In this respect, psychiatry is roughly in the position of physical medicine in 1900. Treatment therefore includes any measures used: (i) to influence the patient's mental state, and (ii) to assist in his or her rehabilitation and return to the community. The measures used comprise the groups shown in Table 5.

Certain measures may be of most value in the acute illness, e.g. physical treatment; others may be of most value in rehabilitation, e.g. industrial therapy. Patients should receive help in as many ways as possible. The acute illness may be controlled by tranquillizers which restore the patient's contact with reality and enable him or her to participate more successfully in psychotherapy, and derive some benefit from a therapeutic environment. Providing the environment is permissive and friendly it is therapeutic rather than antitherapeutic. Social forces too, are important in colouring illness and adding features which are neither symptoms nor signs of illness but merely behaviour patterns imposed by the environment. Violent behaviour has become less common since this was realized. The struggling patient brought into hospital and hurled into a padded room, isolated in total darkness, would be less than normal if he or she did not react in a hostile fashion towards his or her surroundings.

It is important to realize that any hospital admission provokes anxiety mainly because of the uncertainty that the patient experiences and also because the patient feels his or her individuality threatened right from the beginning by

Table 5 Measures used in the treatment of psychiatric illness

Type of illness	Treatment	Use of treatment
Psychological	Psychotherapy Behaviour therapy	Used to deal with individual's symptoms, illness and personality
Physical	Pharmacologic agents, e.g. sedatives, tranquillizers and antidepressant drugs	Used in acute psychoses, depressive illness and 'maintenance' treatment of chronic illness
Occupational	Occupational therapy	Used to divert, stimulate, entertain and encourage the patient's activity and interest
	Industrial therapy	Plays an important part in rehabilitation by giving the patient the chance to work and earn in a sheltered environment

simple things like having to undress and get into bed. After this, much that goes on in hospital seems to reinforce the feeling of isolation and lack of identity so that if the atmosphere is worsened by heightened uncertainty, tension and suppressed violence—all of which can be commonplace in a badly run psychiatric ward—one soon has all the ingredients for a situation of the sort which Kafka has described in such frightening fashion.

Future planning of district psychiatric services in England and Wales should help considerably towards finally removing the stigma and general unease that surround mental hospital admission. The psychiatric unit in a general hospital, working in close cooperation with local services, should provide the best way to use hospital admission without damaging the patient.

Psychological treatment

Individual psychotherapy

Psychotherapy is treatment based on verbal communication between patient and doctor and the formation of a therapeutic relationship between them.

The simplest form, and the most widely practised, is *supportive psychotherapy*, in which the patient is encouraged to talk freely about him or herself and symptoms and problems without exploring his or her unconscious mental life. No attempt is made to give the patient insight about the possible origins of his or her difficulties. The patient's defences are shored up rather than broken down.

Psychoanalysis is the most important type of analytic psychotherapy. The term 'psychoanalysis' is used in two main ways; first it refers to a form of psychotherapy, and second it gives the name to the school of psychology founded by Sigmund Freud.

Psychoanalytic theory is a theory of personality structure and development which stresses the fundamental importance of childhood experience in forming the personality. Freud based his theory on observations made on patients he had treated. Classical Freudian theory has been modified by his followers but the central hypothesis is that human behaviour is determined predominantly by unconscious forces and motives springing from primitive emotional needs, rather than by reason.

In psychoanalysis the analyst seeks to explore and modify the personality structure of the patient by intensive and prolonged exploration of this unconscious mental life. This is achieved by use of the technique of *free association*. The patient lies on a couch and allows his or her thoughts to wander in any direction—in this way dredging up unconscious material of which he or she has previously apparently been quite unaware. The reason for getting the patient to lie down is to cut down to a minimum visual stimuli which might be a distraction. The analyst interprets to the patient the symbolic meaning of his or her dreams and fantasies, in this way helping him or her towards self-insight. It is necessarily a prolonged and time-consuming process.

The most suitable subjects are people with above-average intelligence and good verbal ability. All psychotherapeutic methods acknowledge the fundamental importance of the relationship that exists between patient and doctor in psychotherapy. This relationship can vary from one extreme to another as the patient invests the doctor with every sort of emotion. The trained psychoanalyst accepts this relationship and handles it as part of the therapeutic process. The patient transfers to the doctor emotions which previously he or she had experienced about key figures in his or her personality development—this is called 'the transference'.

Transactional analysis looks at the *modus operandi* of the patient. It teases out the defective understanding, maladaptive response or other unhelpful exchange inherent in the patient's system of behaviour. It may therefore be very helpful to work with the psychiatric social worker and the family in a group. Family therapy is a valuable resource that a good social worker can offer. The family dynamics is an important diagnostic tool.

In therapy the doctor's most important tool is his or her own personality. It thus behoves the doctor to understand him or herself well if this tool is to be sharply honed and used effectively.

Analytic psychotherapy short of full-scale psychoanalysis is commoner and less cumbersome a process, and tends to be concerned with more clearly defined goals such as:

1   resolution of conflict;
2   working through problems and viewing them in a different light; and
3   the relief of pent-up feelings.

A personal analysis is considered necessary training for the psychoanalyst. A non-analytic psychotherapist gains a great deal from a personal analysis but if this is not possible the good psychotherapist needs to be intelligent, intuitive, patient and above all, flexible.

Individual psychotherapy does not end with psychoanalysis. In fact, psychoanalysis is probably the least commonly practised form of psychotherapy, since it is time-consuming and uneconomical. On the other hand, most psychotherapies owe a good deal to psychoanalytic theory without acknowledging it. In recent years there has been a move away from the 'classic' psychoanalytic type therapy towards briefer psychotherapies. Some concentrate on the meaning of the symptom, i.e. 'what sort of help is this patient *really* asking for?' Others pay particular attention to the ('here and now') situation, moving the patient all the time towards solving a particular problem in his or her life that he or she appears to be avoiding. Some psychotherapies are directed at the patient in a way that does not seem explicit but which moves the patient towards independence and self-reliance. Other psychotherapies are existential not only in following existential philosophy, but also in practical terms in that they encourage the patient towards responsibility for the self and one's actions, at the same time helping the patient to look at him or herself as a person in the world and to achieve some understanding of the meaning and significance of his or her existence.

Group psychotherapy

In group therapy the main focus of interest is on the interrelationships within the group, rather than on the highly personal relationships as in individual therapy.

Problems are shared in the group situation, and patients are able to see their own difficulties in inter-personal relationships reflected in the group, and so in a different light. Also they are subject to criticism, encouragement and support from other members of the group.

In practice groups should be small—about twelve members being the ideal number. It is found useful to select members of similar ages and with equal division of sexes. The therapist sits with the group and topics are discussed freely. The therapist adopts a non-directive role, avoiding domination or direction of the group but preventing it from straying into defensive irrelevancies.

Patients do 'psychological work' on their problem but often work is avoided in a variety of ways well described by Yalom (1987). Remaining silent is a common way of avoiding work, as is talking about irrelevancies such as the weather. The therapist's skill is to use techniques to harness the anxiety of the group to produce the performance of psychological work. Insufficient anxiety leads to little pressure for work which is why non-direction and the building of a little tension in silences improves group performance. As trust builds up in a group, *cohesion* between its members further encourages psychological work on individual problems.

Why is group work increasingly popular? Unfortunately perhaps for some patients, the world is not populated by nice nurses or patient doctors who will sit and listen to their woes. It is inhabited by much more awkward folk such as spouses, parents, siblings, children, neighbours and so on, who have their own fish to fry. This is the world the patient has to return to and which is more accurately modelled by the group than individual consultations with a doctor. If the patient can learn the social skills and confidence to share his or her problem in the group, he or she may not only get better, but may also learn how to *prevent relapse* in future by talking to his or her family, friends and neighbours. Another powerful effect of groups is the 'judge and jury' effect. Just as a prisoner in the dock can dismiss a presiding judge as ignorant of the real world of poor backstreets, but cannot ignore the verdict of a jury of his own 'mates', so a patient may dismiss the doctor's remarks but he cannot so easily dismiss a fellow member saying 'And if I were your wife, I'd walk out on you too'. It also has to be said that group therapy, besides being effective (Bovill 1985), is very economical.

Abreaction

This name is given to a therapeutic process in which the patient relives an important past experience which has contributed significantly to the development of his or her illness. The re-enactment is accompanied by discharge of pent-up feeling. Freud found this happening to his patients, particularly under hypnosis, and he reasoned that it would be valuable to induce such states so that the patient would benefit by the emotional discharge. The technique of abreaction is used mainly in acute conversion hysteria precipitated by traumatic events, e.g. wartime disasters. Various methods other than hypnosis have been used to bring about a state of altered consciousness conducive to abreaction.

The most widely used is the slow intravenous injection of a 5% solution of sodium amytal.

Cognitive behaviour therapy

This the general name given to a relatively recent form of psychological treatment. Behaviour therapy has its roots in behaviouristic psychology as opposed to psychotherapy which is founded on dynamic psychology.

Behaviouristic psychology explains human behaviour in terms of stimulus–response mechanisms. Behaviour is regarded as learnt by Pavlovian conditioning processes governed by such processes as drive reduction. Thus neurotic behaviour is simply explained in terms of maladaptive behaviour rather than being linked with complicated intrapersonal emotional development.

It follows from this view of neurotic illness that if the neurotic symptom is removed, the illness disappears too—an entirely opposite view to the psychodynamic one which sees symptoms as symbolic representations of internal conflict. A behaviouristic explanation of a phobic anxiety state would be that the patient has become conditioned to experience anxiety whenever he or she perceives certain signals and that this conditioned response has gradually generalized so that it is triggered off by a wide variety of signals. Behaviour therapy seeks to eradicate the maladaptive response by a process of desensitization.

An individual's patterns of thinking influence behaviour and feeling and thus, by a series of rationally determined procedures, it should be possible to alter abnormal behaviours and feelings. Treatment, therefore, cannot be simply Pavlovian but should contain a cognitive, explanatory element. As well as accelerating recovery, this encourages compliance with treatment by increasing motivation (see, for example, p. 60).

Physical treatment

Nowhere is empiricism more evident than in the sphere of physical treatment in psychiatry. Methods have appeared; a remarkable array of drugs is on the market; all are greeted with initial uncritical enthusiasm and later more soberly evaluated. The whole question of the use of physical treatments has aroused strong feelings on both sides. Nevertheless, it is a fact that certain physical treatments have established themselves as important therapies which have revolutionized psychiatry.

Psychotropic drugs

Psychotropic drugs alter feeling, perception, behaviour or consciousness. The study of such drugs, i.e. psychopharmacology, has not only produced a large range of drugs used in treatment but has also suggested possible lines of research in the biochemistry of mental illness. The *cerebral amine* theory of depression is a good example. According to this theory the central transmitting amines are linked to depression in that it appears that depression can be associated with a low concentration of amines and mania with excessive concentrations. The amines concerned are noradrenaline, serotonin and dopamine. The tricyclic antidepressants are thought to act by blocking the

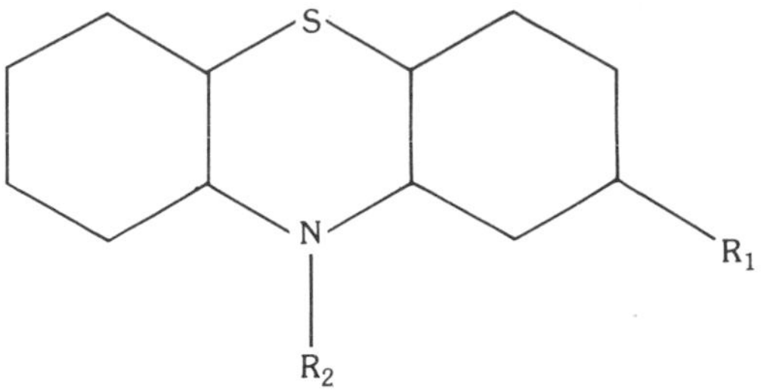

Fig. 8 The structure of phenothiazines.

reabsorption of free amines and the monamine oxidase inhibitors to act by preventing oxidative deamination, in either case causing higher amine concentrations.

The important psychotropic drugs include neuroleptics, antidepressants, tranquillizers and lithium salts.

Neuroleptics and tranquillizers

Tranquillizers are drugs which alter behaviour with minimal impairment of consciousness. Their place in psychiatry dates from 1953 when the tranquillizing effects of *chlorpromazine* were first demonstrated. Chlorpromazine was the first of the phenothiazines to come into use, and the majority of tranquillizers in present use belong to the phenothiazine series. Phenothiazines all have the basic structure shown in Fig. 8, where R_1 and/or R_2 are side chains varying from one phenothiazine to another.

Chlorpromazine (Largactil) is most useful in calming psychotic excitement whether organic, affective or schizophrenic in origin. It is widely used in the maintenance treatment of chronic psychotic patients, but the usefulness here is much less certain. It can be administered by either the intramuscular or the oral route. *Dosage* is up to a maximum of 600 mg per day in divided doses, though a maximum of 400 mg per day is rarely exceeded. The most serious *side-effects* include anaemia, agranulocytosis and jaundice. Less important effects include hypotensive attacks, photosensitivity and dermatitis. Chlorpromazine potentiates the action of barbiturates, alcohol, anaesthetics and narcotic drugs.

Haloperidol is particularly effective in treating the motor overactivity of mania and schizophrenic excitement. Dosage is from 5–100 mg daily depending upon severity. Long-acting intramuscular oily solutions are available and careful intravenous injection is helpful in acute delirium tremens. It is not a phenothiazine, but has similar indications.

Thioridazine (Melleril) has a similar dosage range to chlorpromazine, and similar actions. It is not as powerful but is less sedating and has fewer side-effects.

Trifluoperazine (Stelazine) is said to have an alerting and antihallucinogenic effect in contrast to the sedative effect of the other phenothiazines. It is widely used in the treatment of both acute and chronic schizophrenic patients. It can be administered parenterally or orally. *Dosage* ranges from 5–40 mg per day in divided doses. There is evidence to suggest that in small doses (3 mg tds) it is useful in the treatment of chronic anxiety states.

Long-acting phenothiazine drugs. Compliance of chronic schizophrenic patients with oral drug treatment is poor. Effective long-acting intra-muscular injections of phenothiazine in an oily base (*depot* preparations) are now commonly used. The most popular are: flupenthixol (Depixol), fluphenazine (Modecate), fluspirilene (Redeptin), pipothiazine (Piportil) and chemical variants of these such as Zuclopenthixol (Clopixol).

Extrapyramidal side-effects do occur and can produce severe dystonic reactions. A common practice is to give anticholinergic medication by injection at the same time as the depot. The patient is given a first test dose of the depot which is followed up with the monthly dose.

Side-effects of phenothiazines

These are most commonly neurological syndromes affecting the exrapyramidal system, and include:

1   motor restlessness particularly affecting the legs (akathisia);
2   facial rigidity
3   increased tonus in all four limbs } Parkinsonian syndrome;
4   persistent tongue protrusion and involuntary mouth movements; and
5   dystonic movements of the head and neck.

These side-effects can be controlled by using anticholinergic drugs, which should, however, not be given as a routine. Patients who have been on long-term phenothiazine therapy may develop the syndrome of tardive dyskinesia. This consists of persistent facial movements, grimacing and tongue protrusion which do not stop if the medication is discontinued.

Antidepressant drugs

Drugs used in the treatment of depression fall into two main groups: (i) the tricyclic series, and (ii) the monoamine oxidase inhibitors.

The first drugs used in the treatment of depression were *amphetamine and its derivatives.* They had the advantage of cheapness and a lack of major side-effects. Unfortunately they are readily abused for entertainment. They are also not effective in severe depression.

The tricyclic series

Table 6 lists the most commonly used tricyclic antidepressants. It appears that tricyclic antidepressants act in various ways; some by inhibiting the reabsorption of serotonin (amitriptyline, imipramine, clomipramine), while others inhibit the reabsorption of noradrenaline (noripramine, protriptyline and nortriptyline).

It is now realized that the half-lives of tricylic antidepressant are such that there is no need to use divided daily doses. Common practice now is to give a once daily dosage at night.

Side-effects of tricyclic antidepressants

A wide range have been reported, of which the more common varieties are listed:

Table 6 Tricyclic antidepressants in common usage

Generic name	Trade name	Daily dose (mg)	Comment
Imipramine	Tofranil	75–200	The first and, to date, the most effective
Nortriptyline	Aventyl	75–100	Mildly stimulant
Protriptyline	Concordin	15–45	Mildly stimulant. Higher risk of tachycardia and cardiac arrhythmias
Iprindole	Prondol	45–90	Mildy stimulant
Amitriptyline	Tryptizol	75–200	Sedative—hence often given in one dose at night
Trimipramine	Surmontil	75–150	Sedative—hence often given in one dose at night
Doxepin	Sinequan	75–150	Sedative, marked anxiolytic action
Dothiepin	Prothiaden	75–100	Sedative
Clomipramine	Anafranil	75–100	Sedative. Bad interaction with alcohol. Useful in obsessional cases
Lofepramine	Gamanil	140–210	Safe, few side effects

1   Cardiovascular: hypertension, *orthostatic hypotension*, palpitations, *tachycardia*, arrhythmias.

2   Anticholinergic: *dry mouth*, nausea and vomiting, *constipation*, urinary delay and retention, difficulty in accommodation, mydriasis, *blurred vision*, sublingual adenitis, sweating.

3   Central nervous system: confusional states, excitement, agitation and restlessness, *insomnia*, paraesthesia and tingling, ataxia, tremor, fits.

4   Skin: general and non-specific; rashes, photosensitivity, urticaria, oedema—especially of the tongue and face.

5   Non-specific side-effects include impotence, *drowsiness*, feelings of *weakness and fatigue, weight gain*, weight loss.

6   Rarer adverse effects include myocardial infarction, heart block, extrapyramidal side-effects, paralytic ileus, depression of bone marrow activity, agranulocytosis, purpura, thombocytopenia, black tongue, gynaecomastia, and testicular swelling, breast enlargement and galactorrhoea, and alopecia.

NB Tricyclic antidepressants are very widely prescribed and it may be asked whether they are being overprescribed. The incidence of side-effects is high and also there is a dangerous level of mortality from cardiac arrest and arrhythmia, in cases of overdose and sometimes in cases of therapeutic dosage. For this reason, they should be used with caution and the time really has arrived when the whole question of the widespread use of tricyclic antidepressant drugs needs to be seriously reconsidered since it is beyond doubt that many people who are not depressed are given these drugs and so exposed to considerable hazard. Not every unhappy person who consults a doctor is necessarily depressed.

The monoamine oxidase inhibitors
The first demonstration of the euphoriant effect of this group of drugs was that INAH, used in the treatment of tuberculosis, made patients euphoric. Since then

a large number of monoamine oxidase (MAO) inhibitors have been developed, probably the most common in use are: isocarboxazid (Marplan), dosage range 15–30 mg tds; phenelzine (Nardil), dosage range 15–30 mg tds; tranylcypromine (Parnate), dosage range 15 mg tds to 15 mg qds.

Side-effects of monoamine oxidase inhibitors
1 Potentiation of barbiturates, alcohol, tranquillizers, opiates and pethidine. For this reason their use presents special hazards in anaesthesia.
2 States of excitement and agitation.
3 Hypotension.
4 Hypertensive crises. These occur in certain patients if they eat foods containing *tyramine*, such as certain cheeses, yeast extracts and broad bean pods. Patients should be warned not to eat these foods. The crises, when they occur, are characterized by severe headache which can simulate subarachnoid haemorrhage.
5 Liver damage. This has been found most commonly in the hydrazine series (phenelzine, isocarboxazid).
6 Other common side-effects include oedema, sexual impotence and failure of orgasm; also dryness of the mouth, blurred vision and constipation.

Combinations of MAO inhibitors and tricyclic antidepressants can be dangerous and are probably best avoided.

General observations on the use of antidepressant drugs
Though they are widely prescribed there is by no means universal agreement either as to their efficacy or mode of action. Controlled trials have revealed conflicting results. On the one hand there are those workers who are convinced that antidepressant drugs exert a specific effect on the supposed depressive process, whilst on the other there are those who claim that the drugs act merely by their sedative effect on anxiety and agitation. It has been pointed out that depression has a high rate of natural remission and that the enthusiasm for effects of antidepressant drugs may be accounted for by this alone. Whatever the facts may turn out to be, one thing seems certain and that is that physicians have become more alerted to depression and its existence as a condition meriting attention and treatment.

Drugs used in the treatment of anxiety
Benzodiazepines have now completely replaced barbiturates and they include:
1 chlordiazepoxide (Librium) 10–40 mg tds;
2 diazepam (Valium) 10–40 mg tds;
3 lorazepam (Ativan) 0.5–2 mg tid; and
4 oxazepam (Serenid) 10–30 mg tds.

Nitrazepam (Mogadon), temazepam (Normison) and triazolam (Halcion) are commonly used as hypnotics for initial insomnia. There is no pharmacological difference between tranquillizers and hypnotics except the time they are taken. Initial insomnia is usually caused by problems during the day so that symptomatic treatment of insomnia without treating the cause is bad practice.

Also, benzodiazepines suppress dreaming and tolerance rapidly develops to the hypnotic effect so that they are quickly useless and destructive of the refreshing quality of sleep. Further, they are alarmingly addictive with a withdrawal syndrome of phobic anxiety. Fortunately, this is readily, easily and economically treatable. (See p. 60.)

Vitamins

Large doses of vitamins of the B group are used routinely (a) in the treatment of delirium tremens; and (b) in the treatment of subacute delirious states. Pyridoxine, B6, is used empirically for pre-menstrual tension.

Electroconvulsive therapy

Electroplexy is a successful treatment yet its mode of action is unknown and in some quarters its use is viewed with suspicion. Speculative theories of a neurophysiologic sort suggest that the convulsion alters the conditionability of an intricate system or that it alters the level of arousal of the central nervous system in some way. Other theorists suggest that in some unknown way it alters the balance of a central mood regulating mechanism. These tend to represent the views of those favouring its use.

Those who are on the whole opposed to its use tend to suggest that it is a form of 'shock' treatment which in a way 'shocks' the patient into altered behaviour as in the past patients were 'shocked' by sudden immersion or being whirled around in revolving chairs. It has also been suggested that it is the sudden loss of consciousness which affects the patient. Nevertheless there is more uniformity of agreement about its usefulness than is the case with drugs. It is particulary indicated in depressive stupor and puerperal psychosis.

As it is considered a hazardous treatment, consent of the patient or a second opinion is required.

Technique

A typical machine gives a 100 V discharge for 1 second. This induces instant loss of consciousness followed by convulsion. Nowadays it is usual to give modified ECT and the practice is to modify it by using intravenous anaesthesia (Thiopentone 200–250 mg in a 5% solution) with a muscle relaxant (Scoline or Brevidil) to prevent injury by violent muscular contractions. Oxygen is used to ventilate the patient, and the convulsion is induced. Recovery of consciousness is rapid, i.e. within 10 minutes, and discomfort is no more than a pin prick in the arm. Atropine 0.6 g is given intravenously with the thiopentone.

Treatment is given twice weekly and the patient assessed between treatments. A course of treatment is not prescribed; it is preferable to stop when the patient is better. One should rarely give more than twelve treatments.

Hazards of ECT

Major
1   Normal anaesthetic hazards.
2   Special cardiovascular hazard, e.g. induction of cardiac arrhythmia.

3 Injury to tongue, teeth, bones (longbones, scapula, crush fractures of vertebral bodies).

Minor

4 Amenorrhoea

5 Headache.

6 Burns.

7 Memory loss.

8 Confusional states.

Psychosurgery

Psychosurgery is now much less extensively practised. The original, rather crude types of leucotomy operation have been replaced by highly modified and restricted surgery aimed at dividing connections between the frontal lobes and the thalamus. Other operations such as cingulectomy have also been used. These types of surgery show the best results when persistent tension is present, particularly if it arises on the basis of a depressive state or in obsessional disorders and rarely in chronic schizophrenia. Surgery, though less widely performed, still has a place in carefully selected cases for the relief of chronic states of tension. As it is an irreversible treatment, consent of the patient and a second opinion are both required.

Occupational treatment

Occupational therapy

For many years it has been realized that work can be a source of diversion to the disturbed patient. Nowadays the occupational therapist has a wide range of activities to offer the psychiatric patient. These include art and craft work which can calm the anxious patient or revive the interests of the retarded depressive. Tasks can be provided for the brain-damaged patient which may afford him some degree of satisfaction and promote recovery.

Also the occupational therapist can assess the limits of such a patient's ability and help to provide him with a suitable environment. In rehabilitation the occupational therapy (OT) department can help to plan a patient's daily round of activity to prepare for the return home by helping him or her to acquire new skills or refurbish old ones. The housewife can be particularly helped in this direction by the provision of a kitchen unit in the OT department. Ideally occupational therapy should be realistic and diverse and as far removed as possible from the traditional picture of basket making or the manufacture of useless ornaments.

Industrial therapy

This is an attempt to provide the patient with a working day, a regular wage and the prospects of working outside hospital. It provides a sheltered working environment for the chronic patient where he or she can learn, practise and gain confidence in new skills.

In many hospitals light assembly work, etc. is done on a contract basis with local firms and after a patient has 'proved him or herself' he or she can then go out to work.

Rehabilitation of chronic patients, particularly chronic schizophrenics, is a difficult task. Patients need graded tasks, much encouragement, careful assessment and supervision. In this the doctor is aided by many people, including:

1   nurses with special training and experience;
2   psychologists; and
3   disablement resettlement officers.

Social measures

The social worker

The social worker occupies a central place in psychiatric practice, bringing to it not only a knowledge of social factors and their importance in the aetiology of illness but also more sophisticated awareness of psychodynamics of social systems, particularly the social unit—the family. The work of the social worker includes such diverse activities as:

1   collection of data;
2   therapeutic intervention in pathological social relations, e.g. a community isolate, a family scapegoat, an alcoholic's spouse, etc;
3   social casework: this is a therapeutic technique in which the social worker helps the patient to handle his or her problems, and relate them to his or her social situation;
4   direct counselling about concrete social problems such as finance, housing, etc.; and
5   prophylaxis of psychiatric disorder, aftercare and follow-up.

The therapeutic community

All hospitals are frightening places for the majority of patients, and mental hospitals are particularly so, since often they tend to be large, gaunt buildings with long, anonymous corridors. In fact, if one were to try and devise a way of making a patient worse, one could hardly improve on traditional mental hospital custodial care, which tended to reduce patients to nameless, lost creatures, with no identity. In fairness to those who worked in such conditions it should be pointed out that they had neither the advantages of the tranquillizing drugs of today nor enthusiastic support except from a few benefactors. It is also incorrect to suppose that 'open door' policies are a twentieth-century phenomenon. They are really an extension of the best of English nineteenth-century psychiatry. Unfortunately, as is often the case, pioneering ideas were forgotten and had to be rediscovered.

The moment anyone enters *any* hospital an attack is made on his or her existence as an individual—the clothes are removed, and he or she is put to bed and becomes another patient. In general hospitals, this matters less since the duration of the stay is short and the experience is soon forgotten. But for the

118 CHAPTER 13

psychiatric patient it can be disastrous, since he or she may be entering hospital for a long stay. Before the importance of social factors in influencing mental illness was generally appreciated, the object was to make the patient conform to a number of arbitrary behavioural standards, often of a fairly absurd sort, as quickly as possible. Authority was hierarchical and not to be defied. This made tension increase and violence more likely.

Patients soon learnt to survive by adapting themselves to numbed acquiescence with consequent loss of initiative and drive, so called 'institutionalization'. This was aided by isolation from visitors and lack of activity.

Belatedly it has been realized that the community in which the patient lives can have either a therapeutic or an antitherapeutic effect, and attempts are now made to produce a hospital environment which preserves the patient's individuality and stimulates him or her to activity and a return to the world outside. Emphasis is laid on freeing the lines of communication between medical and nursing staff and encouraging free discussion between patients and staff, thus removing artificial and meaningless barriers. Of course, running hospitals in this way means more work and more trouble as opposed to the apparent calm of a traditional, 'well run' hospital supervised by a superintendent delegating authority downwards. It means more work, but less misery and more hope. Psychiatric patients need hope, noise, colour and activity. Too often their lives can be spent in a grey silence. Anyone who can prevent this is performing a therapeutic act.

References
Bovill, D. (1985) *Tutorial Psychotherapy*. MTP, Lancaster.
Yalom, I. D. (1987) *Group Psychotherapy*. Basic Books, New York.

Further reading
Bloch, S. (1986) *An Introduction to the Psychotherapies*. Oxford University Press, Oxford.
Illich, I. (1975) *Medical Nemesis*. Calder & Boyars, London.
Minuchin, S. (1979) *Families and Family Therapy*. Tavistock, London.
Tennent, T. G. (1980) *Current Trends in Treatment in Psychiatry*. Pitman, London.

Index